Oncology: An Introduction for Nurses and Healthcare Professionals

Oncology: An Introduction for Nurses and Healthcare Professionals

David O'Halloran
Specialist in Cancer Education & Training
Director, O'Halloran Consultancy
Formerly Senior Lecturer in Radiotherapy
School of Healthcare Studies,
University of Leeds, Leeds, UK

ELSEVIER

Notices

Practitioners and researchers must always rely on their own experience and knowledge in evaluating and using any information, methods, compounds or experiments described herein. Because of rapid advances in the medical sciences, in particular, independent verification of diagnoses and drug dosages should be made. To the fullest extent of the law, no responsibility is assumed by Elsevier, authors, editors or contributors for any injury and/or damage to persons or property as a matter of products liability, negligence or otherwise, or from any use or operation of any methods, products, instructions, or ideas contained in the material herein.

ISBN: 978-0-323-88081-7

Content Strategist: Robert Edwards
Content Project Manager: Fariha Nadeem
Design: Patrick Ferguson
Illustration Manager: Nijantha Priyadarshini
Marketing Manager: Deborah Watkins

Printed in India
Last digit is the print number: 9 8 7 6 5 4 3 2 1

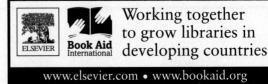

Working together to grow libraries in developing countries

www.elsevier.com • www.bookaid.org

Contents

Preface

Almost 20 years on from the publication of *Notes on Anatomy and Oncology*, the general sentiment of its need persists, which has prompted this re-write. Much has changed in this time, not least our knowledge of cancer and how this knowledge has given rise to many exciting new treatments and treatment strategies. Although given a new title, *Oncology: An Introduction for Nurses and Healthcare Professionals* is an update of the first publication and draws upon much of what is great about the first edition.

I still believe probably more than ever that there is an overwhelming need for those working within cancer services to understand about cancer as a disease. With the ever-changing knowledge base and treatments for cancer, it is important that we keep up to date with our cancer knowledge. Our colleagues expect it, and our patients with cancer deserve it.

Oncology: An Introduction for Nurses and Healthcare Professionals is still written in a way that nonclinicians can understand. It is still a great resource for those new to cancer services or indeed for those who want to update their understanding of cancer and its treatments. It still brings together anatomy and oncology, something that I have not seen any other text do. Having taught about cancer for over 30 years, I feel this combination continues to be essential in understanding cancer. Often the signs and symptoms of cancer are related to the anatomy of the organ of origin. Often, disease progression and metastases will be influenced by relational anatomy, and 'staging', in particular, involves the anatomical extent of the tumour. Without anatomy alongside the oncology, it is difficult for the uninitiated to understand these things. This book continues to bridge this gap and for this reason alone is a very useful reference text.

So, what is new...well, this book reflects the advances in cancer knowledge. Many cancers are driven by specific mutations in key genes which change the way a cancer cell behaves. These 'genetic fingerprints', as I call them, allow us to stratify cancers into smaller, more specific variants. Take lung cancer, for example. It is not good enough to talk solely about lung cancer – we want to know if it is EGFR positive or demonstrates mutated KRAS (read the book to find out what these are!). Such knowledge is allowing for a more targeted treatment strategy leading to a more personalised approach to our treatments and ultimately improving the outcome for these patients.

We have known for a long time that our immune system detects many cancer cells and destroys them. But, of course, some cancer cells persist. Our understanding of how cancer cells may remain undetected has gained ground, leading to the knowledge around 'immune checkpoints' and, as a result, the development of 'checkpoint inhibitor' drugs. Also, the role of T cells in immune detection has allowed for the development of treatments like CAR(T). Utilisation of the immune system to fight cancer is not new, but it has now been taken to a new, and very exciting, level.

Oncology: An Introduction for Nurses and Healthcare Professionals, as with the original version, is not meant to make you an expert in cancer; rather, it covers the science of the disease in a way that is easily accessible. It will provide examples of how to communicate complex information to your peers and patients alike in a way that they can understand. If specialists in the field of cancer find the information in this book useful, then I am honoured. However, this book is not primarily aimed at such professionals as there are many other, more specialised works on the market that will suit their needs. Years of teaching those from a non-cancer, non-academic or science background has allowed me to tailor my teaching, bringing across this information in an understandable way. *Oncology: An Introduction for Nurses and Healthcare Professionals* is the fruit of this experience and will be essential reading for those struggling to get to grips with cancer and its terminology and can be used as a handy tool for comprehending and contextualising the information that you read daily.

Acknowledgements

I understand that no small group of people can have expertise in all branches of oncology. While attempting to bring together my combined years of experience in clinical, academic and private settings, I have been privileged to meet many people – not least of all clinical coders, multi-disciplinary team coordinators, clinical audit staff, medical secretaries, researchers, cancer managers, charity-based staff, clinical trials personnel and others (you know who you are!) – from whom I have learnt a great deal and which has helped me put this manuscript together. Thank you.

Also, although not involved in this update, it is important to mention the contribution of Kathryn Guyers and Jill Henderson on the publication of the initial text, *Notes on Anatomy and Oncology*. I hope this update conveys the same intention and spirit.

Thanks go again to Elsevier, who once again have seen fit to support this endeavour.

No text, book or article can be written without the support and encouragement of those around. I thank all those who have supported me in the work I do and my life in general – you make my world a much brighter place.

Leeds 2023
David O'Halloran

Cells, Tissues and Cancer

Chapter Outline

Objectives

By the end of this chapter the reader should be able to:

- Understand why cancer can be found in many places of the body.
- Relate different cell types to different types of cancer.
- Understand why cancer can move and grow away from the primary site of origin.
- Outline the methods of spread such as local invasion, lymphatic and blood spread, seeding and transcoelomic spread.
- Explain how disease progression will influence patient management.
- Describe how tumours can be classified with specific consideration of staging and grading systems.
- Outline what the likely treatment options are for a patient with cancer

With over 200 different types of cancer in existence, finding one simple definition for this disease is understandably difficult. There are, however, some important similarities among all cancers that together begin to build a picture of what the disease is. In 2000, Hanahan and Weinberg published their seminal paper 'The Hallmarks of Cancer' in the *Cell* journal. Here, they outlined six traits that appear to be common among all neoplasms:

- Cancer cells stimulate their own growth.
- They resist inhibitory signals that might otherwise stop their growth.
- They resist their programmed cell death.
- They can multiply indefinitely.
- They stimulate the growth of blood vessels to supply nutrients to tumours.
- They invade local tissue and spread to distant sites.

In 2011, they proposed two further characteristics:
* Cancer cells have abnormal metabolic pathways.
* They evade the immune system.

These characteristics are generally regarded as present only in abnormal cells. To understand these features of abnormal cells and to subsequently understand how cancer forms and develops, it is necessary to take a look at what makes up a normal cell within the human body.

The Cell

The cell is the basic unit of life, a building block of the human body. Each cell is surrounded by a membrane that separates it from other cells and from the external environment (Fig. 1.1). Known as the plasma membrane (or cell membrane), it acts as the cell's contact with its outside world and allows messages from this external environment to enter the cell. On the surface of the cell there are many receptors, such as the epidermal growth factor receptor (EGFR) (Fig. 1.2), waiting to receive these messages. These are transported by a ligand, or messenger, such as epidermal growth factor (EGF). The ligand binds to the receptor and delivers the message, which is then transported to the nucleus of the cell via a series of specialised proteins called proto-oncogenes (e.g. Ras and Raf). Such transmission of the message is referred to as signal transduction. The message is interpreted by the DNA and the cell responds appropriately. The message might communicate to the cell to continue with its function, to stop doing its function or, indeed, to die (apoptosis). The message might also communicate to the cell the need to divide (mitosis) and produce another cell. Table 1.1 gives some examples of ligands and receptors that are important for cell survival.

The relationship between the ligand and the receptor and the process by which the message is brought

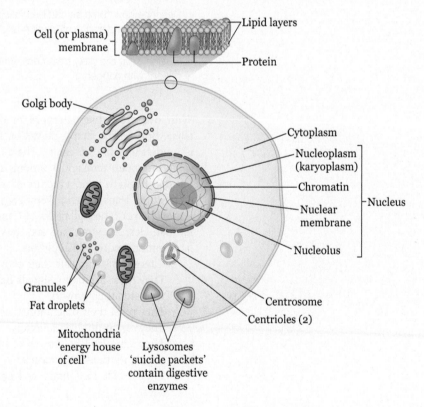

Fig. 1.1 Diagram of cell.

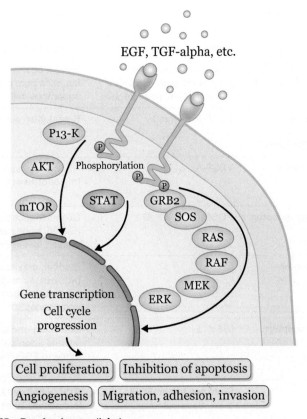

Fig. 1.2 Surface cell receptors. *TGF-α*, Transforming growth factor-α.

to the nucleus is an important process that is disrupted when cancer develops. An understanding of these signalling pathways is crucial to understanding the hallmarks of cancer as outlined above. This knowledge is also necessary for grasping how some of the more modern treatments (targeted therapies) work. More will be said about these signalling pathways later.

The Nucleus

Central to the control and functioning of the cell is the nucleus, which is responsible for cell growth, metabolism and reproduction. The nucleus is usually a round or oval organelle bounded by a membrane called the nuclear membrane. It is the largest structure in the cell. Changes to the shape and size of the nucleus are known as nuclear pleomorphism and may indicate that the cell is undergoing neoplastic change. Within

the nucleus is a nucleolus containing chromosomes, of which there are 46 (23 pairs) in a (diploid) human cell.

While chromosomes are complex, they are basically composed of proteins and DNA, the latter of which carries genetic information and the blueprint for protein synthesis. Genes determine the characteristics of the cell and are the building blocks that make up the chromosomal DNA chains, arranged in a specific sequence on the chromosomes. Chromosomes also control cell structure, direct many of the cells' activities and contain all the genetic material essential for life.

It might be useful to think of the chromosome as a giant recipe book and a gene as a recipe, to make a cake for example. Following the recipe and using the required ingredients results in a (near) perfect cake. If the amount of one of the ingredients is changed slightly, 150 g of flour instead of 225 g, the resulting

TABLE 1.1   Ligands and Receptors Associated With Cancer

Receptor	Ligand (Growth Factor)	Associated Cancer
Epidermal growth factor receptor: EGFR (also called HER1 or ErbB1)	Epidermal growth factor, transforming growth factor alpha (TGF-α), amphiregulin	Breast, bowel, lung, brain, prostate, ovarian, stomach, pancreatic, head and neck squamous cell carcinoma (HNSCC), anal
Human epidermal growth factor receptor 2: HER2 (also called neu, EGFR2, ErbB2)	No known ligand	Breast (also some ovarian, stomach, uterine)
Vascular endothelial growth factor receptor: VEGF-R	VEGF-A, -B, -C, -D	Any cancer with a blood supply. VEGF-R is on endothelial cells lining blood vessels
Platelet-derived growth factor receptor: PDGF-R	PDGF-A, -B, -C, -D	Gliomas, gastrointestinal stromal tumours (GISTs), bone metastasis from prostate cancer; also implicated in angiogenesis
Fibroblast growth factor receptor: FGF-R 1,2,3,4	FGF	Bladder, cervical, multiple myeloma, prostate, small cell lung cancer, breast cancer, stomach cancer; also important in angiogenesis
Insulin-like growth factor-1 receptor: IGF1-R	IGF-1, 2	Bowel, prostate, breast and lung; strongly inhibits apoptosis; associated with resistance to EGF-R inhibitors and chemoresistance
(c-)KIT	Stem cell factor (SCF)	GIST, small cell lung cancer, acute myeloid leukaemia, T cell lymphoma, testicular germ cell, melanoma
Fms-like tyrosine kinase 3: FLT3	FLT3 ligand	Acute myeloid leukaemia
MET	Hepatocyte growth factor (HGF)	Kidney, non-small cell lung cancer, liver, pancreatic, prostate and bone metastasis; important in invasion and metastasis; associated with resistance to EGF-R inhibitors and VEGF-R inhibitors

cake will look different. If something else is changed, the end product looks different again. The more changes that occur result in the end product looking very different to the intended.

Imagine a gene (recipe) which is responsible for producing a protein that promotes cell growth and division in the normal cell. The 'recipe' is important and produces just enough protein to produce 'just enough' cell growth and division. If the gene is changed or mutated, it may produce too much of this growth protein, causing more cell growth and division than intended. More changes and mutations can eventually cause the gene to produce more and more of the proteins, leading to greater and greater cell growth and division. This 'proto-oncogene' (the normal version of the gene) has been transformed into an 'oncogene', a gene now capable of promoting uncontrolled cell growth and division. More will be said about oncogenes later.

The Cell Cycle

During a human lifetime, millions of cells are produced, and millions are lost as cells are damaged, destroyed or die. New cells are constantly needed to replace those that have been lost. It is estimated that in 2 hours 4 million red blood cells die and 4 million grow to replace the lost cells. To maintain the normal balance of cell numbers, cells must go through a cycle (Fig. 1.3) that consists of duplicating every component of the cell along with the chromosomes and results in the division of two identical daughter cells.

Cells with a nucleus are referred to as eukaryotes. A eukaryotic cell cycle can be divided into two stages: interphase and mitotic (M) phase. During interphase, the cell grows, accumulating nutrients needed for mitosis (cell division), and DNA is replicated. In the M phase, the cell splits itself into two daughter cells; these will then enter interphase to begin the process again.

Interphase allows the cell time to gather the nutrients, produce the proteins it needs to enter mitosis and produce another cell. It is a phase of preparation, in which a series of changes takes place making the cell capable of division once again and is subject to various checks and balances. Two such checks and balances are referred to as the G1/S and G2/M checkpoints and are crucial for the progression (or not) of cells through the cycle. For mutated, malignant cells to progress, they must work a way around these checkpoints, and more will be said about this later. Typically, interphase lasts for at least 90% of the total time required for the cell cycle and can be divided into three consecutive phases: G1, S and G2 (Table 1.2).

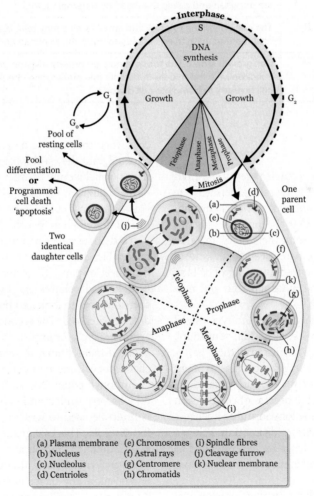

(a) Plasma membrane	(e) Chromosomes	(i) Spindle fibres
(b) Nucleus	(f) Astral rays	(j) Cleavage furrow
(c) Nucleolus	(g) Centromere	(k) Nuclear membrane
(d) Centrioles	(h) Chromatids	

Fig. 1.3 Diagram of cell cycle and cell phases.

TABLE 1.2	Phases of the Cell Cycle		
Phase	**Description**		**Description**
Resting	Gap 0	G_0	Once a cell has undergone mitosis, it may leave the cell cycle and enter G0, a resting phase, carrying on with the normal functions required by that particular cell. It may remain in this phase for long periods of time, possibly indefinitely (as is often the case for neurons), and is common for cells that are fully differentiated. Some cells, such as hepatocytes (liver cells), enter the G0 phase semi-permanently. Others do not enter at all and continue to divide, such as epithelial cells.
Interphase	Gap 1	G_1	The 'initial growth phase'. Internal activities of the cell increase in rate. The cell increases its supply and production of proteins and cellular organelles and grows in size. The G_1 checkpoint control mechanism ensures that everything is ready for DNA synthesis.
	Synthesis	S	The S phase is completed quickly. DNA is unwound and subsequently replicated. During DNA replication, the base pairs (cytosine, thymine, guanine and adenosine) are exposed and easily damaged by external factors
	Gap 2	G_2	The cell continues to grow and small repairs may take place. The G_2 checkpoint ensures that everything is ready to enter the M phase and divide.
Cell division	Mitosis	M	Cell growth stops. The focus is now on orderly division into two daughter cells. A checkpoint in the middle of mitosis (the metaphase checkpoint) ensures that the cell is ready to complete cell division.

Normal Cell Division

Mitosis is a process whereby a single parent cell duplicates itself. It ensures that the two daughter cells are produced with the same number of identical chromosomes as the parent cell. After the process, the two daughter cells possess the same hereditary material and genetic potential as the parent cell. This kind of cell division results in an increased number of cells so that dead and injured cells can be replaced and new cells added for body growth.

Ultimately, the cell will mature into the type of cell it is intended to be, a process called 'differentiation'. Differentiation is a term that is familiar to all those working in the cancer field, where malignant neoplasms might be described as either 'well' or 'poorly' differentiated.

Cells produced through the process of cell division are built in a slightly immature format, and so a process of maturation (differentiation) needs to occur. When a cell has fully matured into the cell it was intended to replace, it is referred to as 'differentiated'. So how does this work with neoplasms?

If, when analysing the cells of a malignant neoplasm down a microscope, they appear similar to normal cells, then they can be described as being well differentiated, and they will look and probably behave like their normal mature counterpart. If, however, the cells of the malignant neoplasms look bizarre and nothing like the normal counterpart (pleomorphic), then they can be described as 'poorly differentiated'.

To demonstrate this further, we can use a sheet of paper (Fig. 1.4). The first sheet of paper (A) is a normal sheet of paper (a normal cell), ideal for printing. It looks and behaves exactly as you would expect a sheet of paper to look and behave: it is a perfect, well-differentiated cell. The second sheet of paper (B), however, is slightly crumpled (a malignant tumour cell). While it looks similar to a normal sheet of paper, the chances of causing a printer jam are significantly higher.

Although paper B is not quite the same as paper A, it looks very similar and is behaving in a similar way. It could be used to write a note or shopping list on, for example. This malignant cell could be referred to as well differentiated because it looks and behaves like its normal counterpart, though it is just not perfect.

The more the paper is crumpled, the less normal it looks. As a small, scrunched-up paper ball (C), it is now as far away from normal as it can be. It is now no

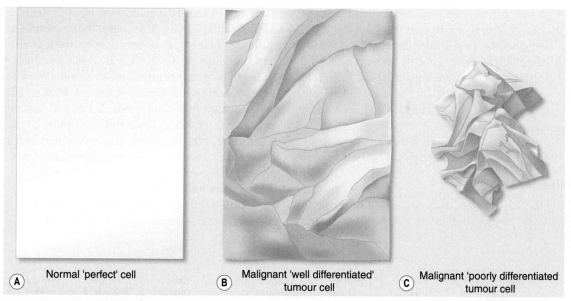

Fig. 1.4 The sheet of paper analogy.

good for printing on or writing a shopping list on; this cell is now poorly differentiated. It neither looks nor behaves like its normal counterpart.

Throwing the normal sheet of paper (the normal cell) results in it not going very far. However, when throwing the crumpled piece of paper (the poorly differentiated malignant cell), it acts more like a ball and goes much further. The poorly differentiated cell does not have the characteristics of the normal cell and has assumed other characteristics; it behaves much better as a missile, for example. It is these new characteristics that will give this poorly differentiated cell the ability to spread (metastasise). From this analogy, it can be seen that there is a link between the level of poor differentiation and the likelihood of metastasis (Fig. 1.5).

The concept of differentiation within a malignant neoplasm is referred to as the 'grade' of a tumour and will be covered in more detail later.

Tissues

Cells of a similar type will group together to form a band of cells that are referred to as a tissue. Tissues wrap around each other to form body organs, which attach to each other to form body systems. These systems work together for the whole body. Such is the level of organisation within the human body.

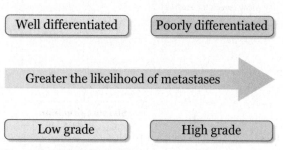

Fig. 1.5 Differentiation and the likelihood of metastasis.

Each specific tissue along with its intercellular substance function together to perform a specific activity, such as protection and support, producing chemicals (enzymes and hormones) or moving food through organs. Tissues can be grouped into several major categories, such as epithelial, connective, muscular and nervous tissue.

DEVELOPMENT OF TISSUES FROM CELL TYPES

There are four basic tissues of the body:

- General supporting tissues, collectively called the mesenchyme: connective tissue, with fibroblasts to form collagen fibres and associated proteins for bone, cartilage, muscle, blood vessels and lymphatic vessels

- Organ-specific cells: epithelium and specific cells for organs such as skin, intestine and liver
- Defence cells: reticuloendothelial cells are a wide group of cells derived mainly from precursor red and white cells in the bone marrow; some cells are also distributed about the body as free cells and others as fixed organs such as lymph nodes and spleen
- Nervous system: central nervous system (brain and spinal cord) and peripheral nervous system

EPITHELIAL TISSUE

Epithelial tissue covers body surfaces (such as skin), lines body cavities and forms glands (Fig. 1.6 and Table 1.3). It forms the outer covering of the body and some internal organs. It also lines body cavities and the inner lining (mucous membrane) of the respiratory tract, gastrointestinal tract, blood vessels and ducts.

Epithelium can be arranged in single (simple) or several (stratified) layers; these cells are held together by specialised fibres and substances (e.g. a basement membrane). Epithelial tissue can be sensitive to stimuli, such as taste and smell, but is avascular (has no blood supply) and receives nutrition by diffusion.

Normal features of epithelial tissue include:

- Closely packed cells
- Little or no intercellular material (matrix)
- Continuous sheets: single or multi-layered

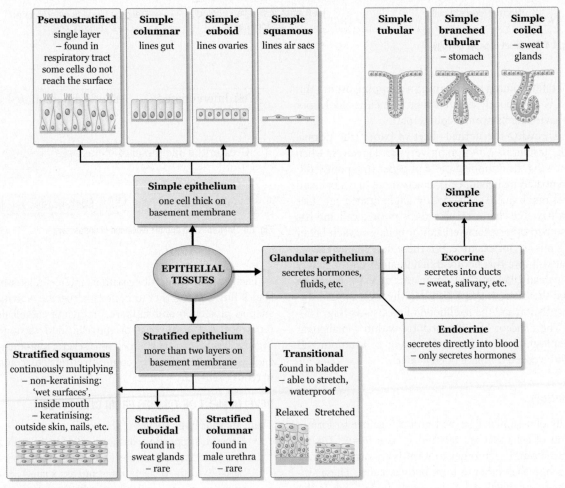

Fig. 1.6 Different epithelial tissues.

TABLE 1.3 Classification of Epithelial Tissue

Epithelial Tissue	Cell Shape	Appearance	Arrangement and Function
Simple	Squamous Cuboidal Columnar	Flat, scale-like, often described as pavement-like cube-like rectangles set on end	Single layers; delicate; found in areas of absorption and filtration; occurs where there is little wear and tear
Stratified	Squamous Cuboidal Columnar Transitional	Same as above A combination of shapes: bottom layer of cuboidal or columnar, middle layer of cuboidal and a superficial layer of cuboidal or squamous epithelium that allows expansion and can be waterproof e.g. bladder	Made of at least two layers that can withstand wear and tear
Pseudostratified	Squamous Cuboidal Columnar	Appears as many-layered cells	Single layer but appears multi-layered; not all cells are in contact with outer surface
Glandular (secretory)	Squamous Cuboidal Columnar	Classified structurally; simple ducts or compound ducts that are branched (e.g. gastric and uterine); coiled tubular (e.g. sweat glands)	Single, or groups of, epithelial cells that function to produce secretions e.g. hormones, saliva, enzymes

- Nerves that may extend through the sheets but blood vessels that do not
- Vessels that supply nutrition and remove waste (blood and lymphatics) lie in underlying connective tissue

Epithelium overlies and closely adheres to connective tissue. The junction between the connective and epithelial tissue is a thin extracellular layer called the 'basement membrane' from which epithelial layers develop. In malignant epithelial neoplasms, penetration of the tumour through the basement membrane (invasion) gives the tumour the potential to spread to other parts of the body. Malignant tumours of epithelial tissue are referred to as 'carcinoma' and then qualified with a prefix to describe further the type of epithelium involved (see the section on 'Classification of Tumours' (p. 24).

Connective Tissue

The many connective tissues of the body are derived from mesenchyme cells which have broken away from the embryonic mesoderm. These mesenchymal cells distribute themselves throughout the three germ layers of the embryo becoming the most abundant tissue in the body. Some remain in an undifferentiated state in the adult, but the majority differentiate into cells that share a number of characteristics, namely, they consist of cells widely scattered within large quantities of an intracellular substance referred to as the extracellular matrix. This extracellular matrix determines the qualities of the tissue for example fluid, semi-fluid or mucoid.

Connective tissue fills the spaces between organs and tissues as well as provides structural and metabolic support for other tissues and organs. The extracellular matrix is made up of fibres in a protein and polysaccharide matrix, secreted and organised by cells. Variations in the composition of the extracellular matrix determine the properties of the connective tissue. For example, if the matrix is calcified, it can form bones or teeth. Specialised forms of the extracellular matrix also make up tendons, cartilage and the cornea of the eye. General connective tissue is either loose or dense, depending on the arrangement of the fibres. The cells sit in a matrix made up of glycoproteins, fibrous proteins and glycosaminoglycan which have been secreted by the fibroblasts. A major component of the matrix is water.

Malignant neoplasms of connective tissues are referred to as 'sarcoma' and are qualified (prefixed) with the type of connective tissue. For example, 'osteosarcoma' is a malignant neoplasm of bone connective tissue. Because of the shared differentiation pathway of connective tissue cells, determining the actual type of sarcoma can be sometimes challenging. Classification of the type of cell along with the matrix is, therefore, essential in determining the respective type of sarcoma.

Connective tissues are defined by three main components: fibres (with the exception of blood), ground substance and cells. All are immersed in the body fluids and can be broadly divided into connective tissue proper, special connective tissue and a series of other, less classifiable types of connective tissues (Fig. 1.7). As the name suggests, connective tissue serves as a connecting system binding all other tissues together. Connective tissue can be categorised as bone tissue,

which includes cartilage, and soft tissue, such as muscular, nervous, fat or fibrous tissue. Its functions are to bind, protect and support organs. Connective tissue has a rich blood supply; in other words, it is highly vascular except for cartilage, which is avascular.

Features of normal connective tissue:

- The cells are widely scattered within large quantities of an intercellular substance referred to as the matrix; the cells of the tissue secrete this.
- The matrix of the tissue determines the qualities of the tissue; for example, fluid, semi-fluid or mucoid.
- Cartilage is a connective tissue, but its matrix is firm and pliable. The matrix of bone is hard and non-pliable.
- The cells also store fat, ingest bacteria and cell debris, form anticoagulants and create antibodies to protect the tissue from disease.

Also, see Table 1.4.

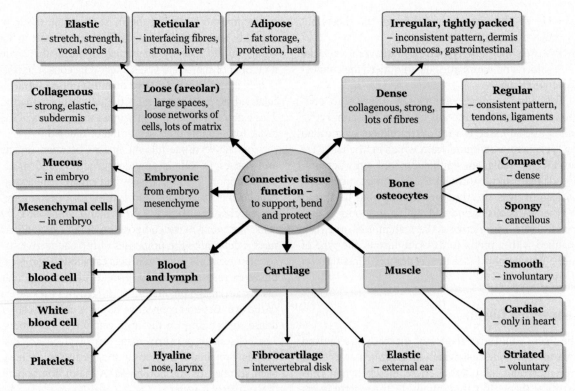

Fig. 1.7 Types of connective tissues.

TABLE 1.4 Epithelial Versus Connective Tissues	
Epithelium	**Connective**
• Covers (skin) and lines (mucosa) • Orderly, cells arranged side by side • Layers of (many) cells • Sensory input, secretion, absorption • Avascular • Innervated (nerves) • High regenerative capacity	• Derived from mesenchyme (embryonic connective tissue) • Most abundant tissue in body • Sporadic cells living in a matrix (water, fibres, collagen) • Protection, binding, support, insulation, transportation • Vascular (except cartilage) • Innervated (except cartilage)

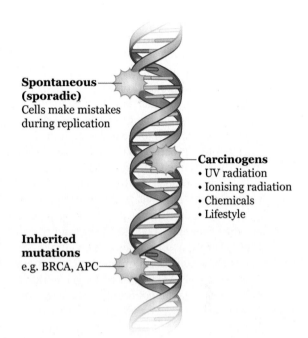

Fig. 1.8 Damage to DNA.

NEOPLASMS

Normal cell replication is under careful control in the body, but sometimes cells will undergo duplication outside the normal control mechanisms of the body. This can result in an excess of new tissue, called a *neoplasm (neo = new, plasm = growth)* or tumour. The study of tumours is called *oncology (onco = mass, bulk; -ology = to study)*. To ensure that a cell is initiated and stimulated through the cycle, there are a number of specialised genes within the cell which will monitor this process. Aberrant or malfunctioning genes may lead to the genetic instability which is the trademark of cancer cells. Such genetic instability will lead to the Hallmarks of Cancer as referred to earlier.

How Do Genes Become Damaged? What Causes Them to Change?

Throughout a lifetime, the human body is exposed to many carcinogens (cancer-causing agents); for example, UV radiation, asbestos, chemicals (benzene) and many others. Such exposure over a long period of time can accumulate damage within the DNA and once again may lead to aberrant cell behaviour which may lead to cancer. Such a progressive accumulation of random damage is why most cancer will appear in people over the age of 50 years (Fig. 1.8).

It is also known that certain damaged genes may be passed on to future generations. The *BRCA 1* and

BRCA 2 genes can be inherited from a person's mother or father. BRCA genes produce proteins which help repair damaged DNA and, therefore, play a crucial role in ensuring the stability of the cell's genetic material. When either of these genes is mutated, or altered, such that its protein product is not made or does not function correctly, DNA damage may not be repaired properly. As a result, cells are more likely to develop additional genetic alterations that can lead to cancer.

ONCOGENES AND TUMOUR SUPPRESSOR GENES

• Proto-oncogenes encourage and promote the growth and division of cells as a response to signals from other cells. This involves relaying information from the cell membrane to the nucleus via the cytoplasm. If these proto-oncogenes are damaged, perhaps by a carcinogen or virus, they can mutate and become oncogenes, which promote the over-production of growth factors and uncontrolled cell growth. Many oncogenes have been researched to date, including, RAS, MYC, HER2 and BRAF. A knowledge of these oncogenes and their role in cancer proliferation and growth has led to a more targeted approach to cancer treatments. Such treatments will be explained later and are designed to inhibit or stop the signal transmissions within the cell (Fig. 1.9).

- *Tumour suppressor genes*, such as *TP53, PTEN* and the Retinoblastoma (*Rb*) genes, act as guardians for the cell, monitoring any mutations. At certain points within the cell cycle, the cell will effectively check itself to see that everything is in order before it proceeds to the next phase of the cycle; these are the G1/S and G2/M checkpoints and will be outlined further when discussing the Hallmarks of Cancer. Tumour suppressor genes are responsible for this checking process and they stimulate apoptosis (programmed cell death) if there is a possibility that cell division may result is some form of mutation. If tumour suppressor genes are lost, or no longer working, and therefore not monitoring for damage, the cell will be allowed to divide, even in a damaged format. Lost or inactivated tumour suppressor genes can be a common prelude to cancer and tumour development. For example, in over 50% of all tumours, the tumour suppressor gene p53 is damaged.

Abnormal cell production may cause an accumulation of too many cells, known as hyperplasia (Fig. 1.10). When this occurs, while there may be an increase in cell numbers, each individual cell appears normal (well differentiated). Hyperplasia is typical in benign neoplasms and may also be accompanied by an increase in the size of the cells (hypertrophy), which is often a response to cell damage or destruction, or increased hormone stimulation.

Metaplasia (meta = change; -plasia = form, growth) may occur because of chronic irritation. Here the cell changes from one type of epithelium to another one

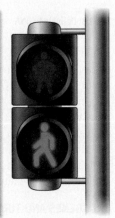

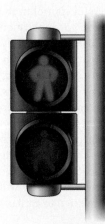

- Proteins from (proto) oncogenes promote cell growth, survival and proliferation e.g. EGFR, RAS, B-Raf, HER2

- In cancer cells oncogenes are overactive, mutated or amplified thereby making too much protein

- Proteins from tumour suppressor genes stop cell growth and replication, may trigger apoptosis e.g. RB, PTEN, TP53

- In cancer cells tumour suppressor genes are lost or not working

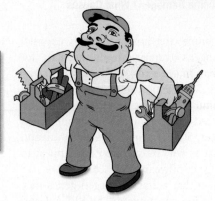

- DNA repair genes sense damage and repair damaged DNA e.g. BRCA; sometimes classed as tumour suppressor genes

- In cancer cells DNA repair genes are lost or not working

Fig. 1.9 (Proto) oncogenes and tumour suppressor genes.

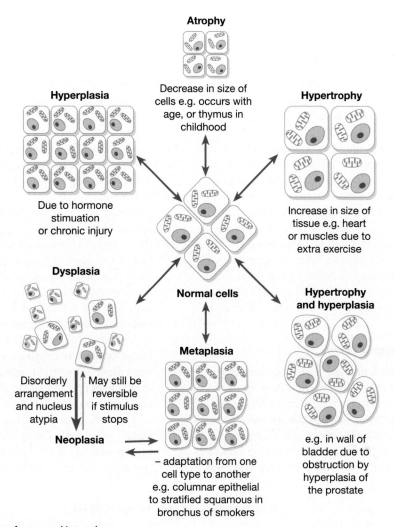

Atrophy

Decrease in size of
cells e.g. occurs with
age, or thymus in
childhood

Hyperplasia

Due to hormone
stimuation
or chronic injury

Hypertrophy

Increase in size of
tissue e.g. heart
or muscles due to
extra exercise

Dysplasia

Disorderly
arrangement
and nucleus
atypia

May still be
reversible
if stimulus
stops

Neoplasia

Normal cells

Metaplasia

– adaptation from one
cell type to another
e.g. columnar epithelial
to stratified squamous in
bronchus of smokers

**Hypertrophy
and hyperplasia**

e.g. in wall of
bladder due to
obstruction by
hyperplasia of
the prostate

Fig. 1.10 Cellular changes from normal to neoplasm.

that can best deal with the irritable environment. For example, metaplasia can be seen in the lungs of smokers where the cells change from ciliated columnar epithelium to stratified squamous epithelium which is more suited to dealing with the chronic irritation. Barrett oesophagus is a condition found in those who suffer from chronic regurgitation of stomach acid into the lower part of the oesophagus. As a result of this chronic irritation, the cells of the lower oesophagus undergo a metaplastic change from squamous to columnar epithelium. Such changes will persist if the irritation continues and may lead to further changes where the cells start to become even more disorganised, leading to dysplasia and neoplasia.

Dysplasia causes more disordered growth than hyperplasia, and the cells may demonstrate changes in cell shape growth or differentiation. Dysplasia restricted to the original tissue is referred to as in situ and by definition is non- or pre-invasive. The concept of in situ will be discussed in more detail later.

Also, note the direction of the arrows between metaplasia/dysplasia and neoplasia in Fig. 1.10. The dual direction indicates that these conditions may be reversible. By stopping smoking, the constant irritation stops and, as such, gives the epithelium a chance to return to normal. If the acid regurgitation is stopped, then, similarly, the lower part of the oesophagus may be able to return to normal. Such interventions can therefore reduce the risk of developing cancer of the lung or oesophagus, respectively.

Cancer Formation (Carcinogenesis)

At times the body will over-produce cells (hyperplasia; see Fig. 1.10) due to normal growth processes; for example, enlargement of the uterus during pregnancy. However, if the stimulus is removed the over-production of cells stops and the cells return to normal. In cancer, however, the cells of the neoplasm (new growth, tumour) continue to divide and grow. Cancer development or carcinogenesis is thought to be a 'multiple hit process' whereby the cell accumulates damage.

The more damaged the cell is, the more likely that proto-oncogenes will mutate into oncogenes that promote cell growth and division. At the same time, tumour suppressor genes can be damaged and become inactivated or lost, which allows mutated cells to continue to divide.

The Progressive Nature of Cancer

Cancer results from a process of genetic change over many years. Cancer is a progressive disease, an accumulation of random damage to our genes which culminates in a neoplasm (*neo-, new; -plasm, growth*). These little bits of random damage occur over a lifetime.

A good analogy might be someone knocking a house down with a toffee hammer! Not an easy task, but imagine someone using the toffee hammer on the bricks and mortar, hammering away every day for 40 years! Little bits of damage here, little bits of damage there. Eventually, the toffee hammer will do so much damage that the house will fall. Imagine little bits of random damage to our DNA over a lifetime–damage that eventually might cause enough change, enough mutation, for cancer to develop! Most cancer occurs in people over the age of 50 years (Fig. 1.11) because of the simple fact that it takes time for this damage to be accrued.

Broadly, the damage that is received can be divided into three groups:

1. Sporadic, Spontaneous Damage

   Or 'bad luck'. Some people just get cancer and there seems to be no real cause as to the changes that must have occurred. In cell replication, there is a doubling up of all cell components, in particular, DNA. DNA is extremely long and complex, and sometimes the process of copying and transcribing DNA goes wrong.

   Imagine being presented with all the Harry Potter books (lucky you!) and your role is to copy them out word for word, day after day, for at least a month. In this 'simple' process of copying these words, you will make mistakes.

   The cell, when copying DNA, sometimes makes mistakes! Often these mistakes can be repaired or, if not, the cell will 'apoptose' (programmed cell death). But sometimes the

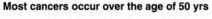

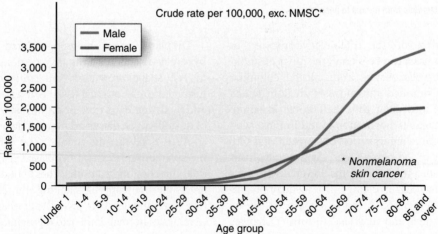

Fig. 1.11 Incidence of cancer by age.

mistakes are not repaired, or it allows the DNA and cell to continue the replication process in a damaged form. This damage is taken into the next cell, then more damage is done, then more, then more....

Such a process might explain why some types of cancer occur. Such spontaneous damage might also be further exacerbated by other types of damage.

2. Exposure to Carcinogens

Carcinogens are 'cancer-causing agents' (or at least potentially cancer-causing). And this exposure can be gained in one of two ways:

Environmental

There are things in our external environment which might be cancer-causing; for example, exposure to car exhaust fumes whilst walking down the street. Such fumes contain carbon dioxide, carbon monoxide and hydrocarbons (amongst other things), which are known carcinogens.

Certain land areas are situated on top of granite rock which can contain naturally occurring radioactive elements such as radium, uranium and thorium. Such elements can decay to produce radon gas, a known carcinogen.

Self-Induced

Appropriate lifestyle choices can limit exposure to some known carcinogens and reduce the risk of getting certain cancers.

Smoking tobacco increases the risk of getting cancer, especially lung cancer. Alcohol and UV radiation from sunlight and sunbeds also increase the risk. There is a known relationship with diet and certain types of cancer and processed meats, and red meat is also cited as containing known carcinogens.

These are just a few examples. But being exposed to these chemicals induces damage within our DNA which can lead to cancer. A person who smokes does not develop lung cancer immediately after starting smoking; it will take years for these changes to take effect, such that most people with lung cancer will be over the age of 55 years.

3. Inherited Damage

Some people may inherit damaged genes (BRCA gene, APC gene) which will pre-dispose them to certain types of cancer. In this unfortunate circumstance, the damage may have already been accrued and passed to the next generation. Lynch syndrome (formerly, hereditary non-polyposis colorectal cancer [HNPCC]) is a rare disorder which can run in families, and people affected by Lynch syndrome have a higher chance of developing various types of cancer including bowel cancer, uterine cancer and ovarian cancer.

This recurring, continuing, relentless damage happens over a long period and is exacerbated in the subsequent generations of cancer cells and carried forward to the next. Cancer is a progressive disease; it takes time to evolve, which is why the majority of people who get cancer are older.

Benign Neoplasms

In benign tumours, there may be few small mutations; the cells will be cytologically identical to their tissue of origin (well differentiated), but histologically they appear as an over-production of cells (hyperplasia; see Fig. 1.10). Benign tumours have a capsule that makes them relatively easy to remove. Benign tumours are not usually fatal. The exception is the pituitary gland, where about 99% of tumours are benign but the site of the tumour (located in the *sella turcica*, a small depression in the bony plate in the base of the skull) is potentially life-threatening. As a pituitary tumour enlarges, the patient displays intracranial pressure symptoms that have fatal implications if not treated.

Malignant Neoplasms

Malignant neoplasms, on the other hand, usually have a central body with infiltrating projections that extend out to invade adjacent tissues. Malignant neoplasms are not held within a capsule but will infiltrate locally and starve the normal adjacent tissue of its blood supply. Malignant neoplasms will eventually break away and spread throughout the body, a process called *metastasis*. Metastatic cells are found in a distant organ and have not developed from the tissue of that organ. For example, if a breast cancer cell is found in the liver, cytologically it will resemble breast tissue. A summary of the differences between benign and malignant tumours is shown in Table 1.5.

Malignancy is defined by the ability to invade local tissue and spread to other parts of the body. Epithelial tissue, as stated earlier, is separated from the connective tissue by a basement membrane and is avascular, meaning it does not have blood or lymphatic vessels within it. Rather, the blood and lymphatic lymph vessels can be found below the basement membrane intermingled with the connective tissues. Epithelial cells obtain oxygen and nutrients, and eliminate waste, via a process of diffusion across the basement membrane.

TABLE 1.5 Differences Between Benign and Malignant Neoplasms	
Benign	**Malignant**
Encapsulated	Not encapsulated
Grow by expansion and never invade. Produce pressure effects or systemic effects and may secrete hormones	Grow by expansion and invasion (direct spread)
Usually slow growing	Growth rate can vary
Under some normal control of body	Under no control
Remain localised	Spread from primary site – metastasise
Cells resemble original tissue; well differentiated	Cells have a variety of presentations from well differentiated to very poorly differentiated (anaplastic)
Not usually fatal, unless pressing on a vital organ	Always fatal unless treated

As a result of damage and irritation, the epithelial cells may undergo metaplastic or dysplastic changes resulting in cells that have cancerous properties. But these cells remain confined by the basement membrane and are said to be in situ. Referring to Fig. 1.12, only epithelial tissue has the potential for this in situ phase, whereas, in contrast, connective tissue is in intimate contact with the blood and lymph vessels and is not separated by a basement membrane. As the cells of the neoplasm continued to receive damage, or progressively mutate, they will begin to develop characteristics, the hallmarks of cancer, that will allow them to invade through the basement membrane. When this happens, the neoplasm is said to be *invasive*. Such a breach of the basement membrane allows malignant cells to further infiltrate the surrounding tissue and potentially spread into the blood and lymphatic vessels. Consequently, the malignant neoplasm can be transported to other parts of the body, meaning it can metastasise.

Tumour Growth

In normal tissue following a mitotic division (see Fig. 1.3), two identical daughter cells are produced. One daughter cell will stay available for cell division (G_0) and one cell will go on to develop into a mature cell with specialised structures and functions. This process where a cell changes and becomes specialised and mature is called *differentiation* and is a normal process that the majority of cells of the body will go through. There are some tissues that maintain the ability to divide throughout life, usually in an area under constant wear and tear that requires a constant supply of newly produced cells such as the lining of

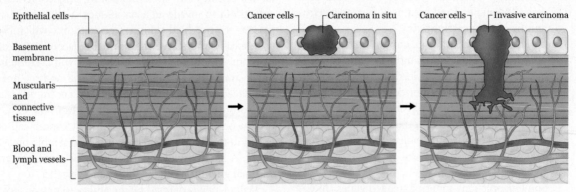

Epithelial cells — Cancer cells — Carcinoma in situ — Cancer cells — Invasive carcinoma

Basement membrane —

Muscularis and connective tissue —

Blood and lymph vessels —

Fig. 1.12 Carcinoma in situ versus invasive carcinoma.

the alimentary tract. As cells become more specialised, they lose their ability to reproduce. Nerve cells are highly specialised and cannot reproduce; tumours of true nerve cells are extremely rare; however, tumours known as gliomas do arise from cells that support the nerve cells called glial cells. Tumour cells, however, tend to divide more frequently than normal cells. Even within a single tumour, the rate of growth – the balance between tumour cell growth and tumour cell death – can vary enormously. This variable mitotic rate can result in different parts of the tumour demonstrating varied differentiation.

Differentiation suggests that the tumour cell looks, and probably behaves, like its parent cell. The less differentiated (poorly differentiated or *undifferentiated*) a cell is, the more mutated it is and the less like the parent tissue it looks and acts. Assessing the degree of differentiation is called *grading* and is defined as '*an estimate of the degree of malignancy*'. Also, a neoplasm's growth depends on its blood supply. A tumour that outgrows its blood supply can develop areas of *necrosis* (death) where cells have been starved of oxygen.

Malignant Tumours and the Hallmarks of Cancer

The ability to metastasise is the fundamental difference between benign and malignant tumours. In most cases, metastasis – rather than the primary tumour – will be the cause of death. As malignant tumours continue to grow and divide, they become increasingly mutated and poorly differentiated. As this happens, they will develop certain characteristics, namely, the hallmarks of cancer. The more poorly differentiated a tumour cell is, the more of these characteristics it will demonstrate, and the more of these characteristics it demonstrates, the easier it will be for it to grow uncontrollably and spread.

HALLMARK 1: CANCER CELLS STIMULATE THEIR OWN GROWTH

Cells of the body are constantly receiving stimuli from the other cells which surround them. In this microenvironment, messages (growth factors) are constantly being exchanged that promote cell growth, replication and survival. Growth factors are responsible for initiating the signalling pathway in cells. This pathway is the cell's method by which it converts an external message into an internal response. On the surface of every cell,

there are receptors waiting to receive a growth factor. Each growth factor will fit and bind to a specific receptor. For a list of receptors and that associated growth factors, refer to Table 1.1.

Receptors are essentially made up of two parts, an external portion, which protrudes out of the cell and allows for the attachment of the growth factor, and an internal portion, which protrudes inside the cell from the membrane. Such an arrangement allows for the growth factor message to be taken inside the cell. The epidermal growth factor (EGF) binds to the epidermal growth factor receptor (EGFR) as shown in Fig. 1.2. What happens next is a process called signal transduction caused by phosphorylation of downstream proteins. When a growth factor binds to a receptor it activates the internal portion. This internal portion, called kinase, transfers a phosphate group to the next protein. Most of the proteins in these signalling pathways work by a simple on/off process. The addition or removal of the phosphate group will switch the next protein on or off. Therefore transferring the message on comprises a simple process of passing the phosphate group to the next protein, then the next, then the next, until it reaches the nucleus of the cell. Here it can affect genes, triggering a cellular response of growth, replication and survival (Fig. 1.13).

In a cancer cell, this signalling pathway seems to be permanently switched on. How does this happen? Essentially, there are three main ways in which the cell escapes the normal signalling pathway.

First, cancer cells are good at manufacturing their own growth factors, which leads to neighbouring cancer cells producing their own growth factors; the whole process is self-promoting. A lot of growth factors mean many signal transductions, which means a lot of cancer cell growth, replication and survival.

Second, cancer cells may have a faulty receptor that is permanently switched on regardless of whether a growth factor is present or not, meaning that the cancer cell's messaging system is always active. The cancer cell may also produce more than the normal number of receptors, causing hypersensitivity to any growth factors present in the tissue and resulting in more cancer growth, replication and survival.

Third, the proteins inside the cell that are responsible for passing on the message internally may also be permanently switched on. Such a situation means that

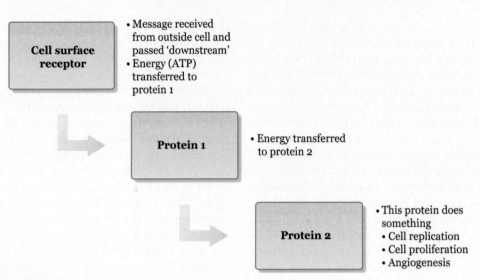

Fig. 1.13 Signal transduction.

the cell does not have to rely on the growth factor, or receptor, as the message will be started inside the cell by a faulty protein. In Fig. 1.2, notice the Ras protein, downstream from EGFR, inside the cell. Mutated or damaged Ras is usually associated with aggressive disease, and poor prognosis and is found in one-quarter of all cancers and over 90% of pancreatic cancers.

Cancer, it would seem, is a consequence of this messaging system being permanently switched on. A strategy to treat cancer then will be to switch off this messaging system in the cancer cell, and this forms the basis of targeted therapy with the three areas mentioned above providing the targets. Inhibitors of these targets stop the message and prevent over-replication and growth of cancer cells. Cetuximab is an example of such an inhibitor and targets the external portion of EGFR, which is overactive, or overexpressed, in many head and neck cancers and colon cancer, and this drug is routinely used in the treatment of these cancers. Identification of suitable targets, and the production of effective inhibitors, will hopefully lead to more effective treatments in the future.

HALLMARK 2: CANCER CELLS RESIST INHIBITORY SIGNALS THAT MIGHT OTHERWISE STOP THEIR GROWTH

As previously discussed, cells must go through the cell cycle to replicate. Made up of phases, the cycle is how

a perfect replica cell is produced and, in particular, DNA is replicated. Throughout this process and before the replicating cell can move into the next phase, there are a series of checks and balances designed to make sure that only a perfect cell along with perfect DNA is allowed to replicate. One especially important monitor is the retinoblastoma protein (pRb).

The role of an active pRb is to bind to the E2F transcription factor and prevent the cell from advancing from the G1 to the S phase of the cycle. It acts as a kind of brake, and in order for the cell to progress, the brake, needs to be released. Therefore the route to progression is simple: disassociate Rb from E2F. The catalyst for this is the cyclin–CDK complex, which phosphorylates Rb and makes it inactive. Inactive pRb detaches from the E2F transcription factor, allowing E2F itself to become active, which effectively pushes the cell into the next phase of the cycle.

Whether or not a cell will progress through the cycle is driven by anti-growth signals. One such anti-growth signal is the TGF-β protein, and its presence halts the progression of the cell cycle. It is the disruption of these pathways that allows cancer cells to continue through the cycle even if it is not ready to do so. Cancer cells may stop responding to the presence of TGF-β and will stop producing receptors so that TGF-β cannot bind on successfully. Alternatively, it will stop or ignore the downstream proteins from

TGF-β, with the net result being that the cell does not receive the anti-growth signal and therefore carries on regardless.

In some cancer cells, the Rb protein is lost altogether. For example, HPV produces a certain protein that binds to Rb and prevents its action. The inability of Rb to do its job either because it is directly inhibited or because it does not receive the message means that damaged cells – cancer cells – are able to replicate unhindered.

Another important antigrowth signal in normal cells is *contact inhibition*. When normal cells are seeded into a Petri dish, they begin to divide and proliferate. As the cells fill the space, they start to touch one another and, consequently, begin to slow their rate of division. Such behaviour is called contact inhibition. Once the space is filled, the rate of cell division becomes balanced with the rate of cell death, resulting in the number of cells remaining the same. Contact inhibition is the body's way of keeping cell numbers constant.

Cancer cells behave quite differently, and when seeded among normal cells, all the cells will proliferate as normal until they fill up the space provided. But where normal cells begin to slow their rate of division because of contact inhibition, cancer cells do not; they lose this inhibitory signal and continue to proliferate in an unregulated manner, yielding a clump of cells referred to as a tumour or neoplasm.

HALLMARK 3: THEY RESIST THEIR PROGRAMMED CELL DEATH (APOPTOSIS)

In normal tissues, a balance must be struck between the number of new cells generated (cell division) and the number of cells lost. Old or damaged cells are constantly being replaced, and like cell division, cell death is also tightly controlled. Programmed cell death, or apoptosis, is the cellular equivalent of a 'self-destruct' button and will be pressed if the cell is too damaged to be repaired.

Apoptosis is an orderly process in which there is an initiation phase and an execution phase. The initiation phase may start outside the cell and consists of a message, or stresses, which signal the cell for destruction; low oxygen levels or radiation damage, for example. Damage inside the cell may also trigger the initiation of apoptosis. Certain treatments like radiotherapy and chemotherapy may damage the DNA sufficiently to kick-start this process. This initiation phase, however triggered, will lead to the execution phase where the activation of a series of specialised enzymes will result in cell death.

The Bcl-2 family of proteins is crucial in controlling the intracellular pathway of cell destruction comprising around 25 different proteins, and this family is responsible for either stimulating or blocking apoptosis. Damage to the DNA, for example, will trigger a cascade of signals which will eventually lead to apoptosis, and it is the Bcl-2 proteins which will initiate this or block this. Certain neoplasms – for example, follicular lymphoma and small cell lung cancer – may over-express anti-apoptotic Bcl-2 proteins. Although this will not directly lead to cancer, it does mean that these mutated cells will not die efficiently and continue to grow and replicate. Mutated or aberrant Bcl-2 is associated with poor prognosis in these neoplasms. These self-destruct proteins are tightly regulated by the tumour suppressor protein p53.

Apoptosis is another of the checks and balances built into the cell cycle, and when something goes wrong, the cell is quickly destroyed. The normal body does not want mutated or damaged cells dividing. If apoptosis does not occur, these damaged cells may survive and develop and therefore plays a crucial role in cancer development and progression. Generally, cancer cells are able to evade apoptosis and the loss of the tumour suppressor gene is a major cause. Such a loss has the consequence that damage within the cell is not picked up, the Bcl-2 family of proteins are not regulated and the cell does not receive the signal to self-destruct. Coupling this with the previous hallmarks where the growth signal is constantly active means damaged cells are able to survive and replicate.

Also, for cancer cells to move to another part of the body (metastasise), they must be able to survive in the blood or lymphatic systems and invade foreign tissue. Loss of contact inhibition means these cells may survive, even though they are not 'touching' other cells. Normally apoptosis would prevent these things.

HALLMARK 4: CANCER CELLS CAN MULTIPLY INDEFINITELY

Generally, cells of the body are allowed only so many cell divisions and then cell division halts. Usually, after around 52 divisions (known as the Hayflick limit) the cell will stop dividing. Such haltering is linked to the 'telomere', an extra length of DNA at the end of the chromosome which protects the DNA from damage which would result in apoptosis. After each cell division the telomere shortens and after around 52 divisions will initiate apoptosis. Such a process means that old cells can be replaced by new ones.

Telomerase is an enzyme which promotes the growth of the telomere and is present in embryonic cells along with some stem cells but is largely absent in adult cells, thereby giving them mortality and only a certain number of cell divisions. Telomerase is present in large quantities in cancer cells which, in effect, rebuilds telomeric DNA and keeps the telomere long and therefore allows cancer cells to continue dividing indefinitely.

It is thought that virtually all cancer cells have this ability to re-build the telomere. An interesting avenue for research to explore would be to work out how this rebuilding could be halted in cancer cells and thereby limit their reproductive capacity.

HALLMARK 5: ANGIOGENESIS; THE FORMATION OF NEW BLOOD VESSELS

As a normal part of growth development and wound healing, the body must grow new blood vessels to oxygenate the tissues. In a process called angiogenesis, new blood vessels sprout from existing ones. On stimulation by angiogenic growth factors, endothelial cells, present on pre-existing blood vessels, break through the basement membrane confining them and begin to proliferate into the surrounding tissues, forming a sprout that will extend towards the angiogenic source. Vascular endothelial growth factor (VEGF) is an active component of this process.

Angiogenesis is a vital process in the development of tumours. A neoplasm needs to grow only to a few millimetres in size before it will become oxygen deficient. As a result, it will begin to send out angiogenic growth factors such as VEGF that will diffuse through the tissues, activating endothelial cells on nearby blood vessels and leading to new blood vessel formation. An understanding of this process is leading to the development of novel targeted therapies designed to inhibit the process of angiogenesis with varying clinical results.

Bevacizumab (Avastin) was the first anti-angiogenic used for the treatment of metastatic colon cancer, and since then other anti-angiogenics have been developed. They work in slightly different ways and target different parts of the angiogenic pathways, but the premise is the same: to stop the formation of new blood vessels and starve the tumour of vital nutrients and oxygen.

However, angiogenesis, as suggested earlier, is a normal and vital process within the human body, and anti-angiogenics have the potential to also disrupt the normal blood vessel formation that is required in the healthy body. Thus, using these drugs to inhibit cancer blood vessel formation may also have a detrimental impact on the normal body.

HALLMARK 6: THEY CAN INVADE AND SPREAD TO DISTANT SITES (METASTASIS)

Epithelial cells stay tightly packed and are joined together through a process of junctions. They are confined by their basement membrane and remain in their locale. It is now known that cancer cells undergo a transformation from epithelial cells to a more primitive mesenchymal cell (Fig. 1.14). Such a transition is called epithelial-to-mesenchymal transition (EMT); mesenchymal cells can disconnect from the

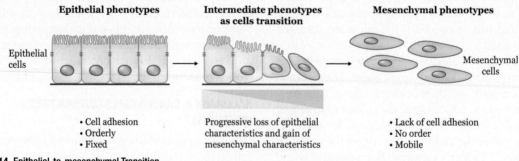

Epithelial phenotypes

Epithelial cells

Intermediate phenotypes as cells transition

Mesenchymal phenotypes

Mesenchymal cells

- Cell adhesion
- Orderly
- Fixed

Progressive loss of epithelial characteristics and gain of mesenchymal characteristics

- Lack of cell adhesion
- No order
- Mobile

Fig. 1.14 Epithelial-to-mesenchymal Transition.

surrounding cellular framework, losing their cellular adhesive qualities and becoming motile. As such, they can disconnect from the basement membrane and interact directly with the connective tissues around the epithelial cells, which is called invasion.

It is worth noting here that cancer cells appear to hijack what is a normal mechanism during human development within the embryo. The human body consists of trillions and trillions of cells and each of these cells have developed from a single blastocyte (a fusion between the ova and sperm). During the process of embryonic development, primitive cells need to be able to migrate to where they are needed and to differentiate into (become) different types of cells. This seems to be exactly what the cancer cells can do.

Bodily tissues consist of primarily epithelial and mesenchymal cells as discussed earlier. Epithelial cells are designed to line the insides and sometimes the outside of body organs, offering protection (mainly) from the outside environment. Mesenchymal cells, on the other hand, are designed to move freely through the intercellular spaces via what is termed the extracellular matrix. Mesenchymal cells are able to differentiate into other types of cells such as bone and cartilage.

Once the cancer cell has migrated to different parts of the body, it may get lodged and continues to grow and divide forming a metastasis. Interestingly, the cells of this metastasis will resemble the cells and tissues from where it originated. For example, a metastasis in the liver that came from a primary breast carcinoma will demonstrate characteristics of the breast cells rather than the liver. Hence, it is further assumed that the cells of the metastasis must undergo the reverse of EMT and transform back into the epithelial type of cells, which is referred to as mesenchymal–epithelial transition or MET.

Further research and understanding of this process will help improve knowledge of the concept of metastasis, and drugs may be developed that can inhibit EMT and/or MET and thus prevent metastasis from occurring. If the cancer can be kept in the locale from where it originated, the primary site, treatment will be much more successful.

METASTASIS: WHY AND HOW CANCER SPREADS

Metastasis, spread and secondaries are all interchangeable terms when it comes to cancer. As a defining characteristic, it plays a major role in how patients are managed and treated. If cancer stayed in the initial locale, its 'primary site', then treatment would be simpler and more successful in most cases. The fact that malignant cells are able to break off and travel to other sites around the body makes treatment more of a challenge. Patients who die of cancer generally die as a result of a 'secondary' tumour, not the 'primary' tumour. This concept of metastasis is crucial to understand.

Cancer cells may spread via several processes, namely, local invasion, lymphatic, blood and transcoelomic (across a cavity).

LOCAL/DIRECT INVASION

Local invasion, or direct spread, refers to the tumour invading the direct vicinity of where it starts. The characteristics of the tumour cells change from being orderly and fixed to losing cellular adhesion, lacking order and becoming mobile. The tumour cells can now invade through basement membranes and other local tissues.

The local invasion can often dictate the signs and symptoms that a person may come through the door with. Skin tumours may destroy tissue, leaving an ulcer-like lesion on the surface of the skin. A person with a lung tumour may present with a productive cough as the tumour invades and destroys local lung tissue. Similarly, someone with a brain tumour may have different signs and symptoms depending on the area of the brain involved. Patients with tumours involving the frontal lobe may become more aggressive, or 'change personality'. A person with bladder cancer may experience bleeding which is picked up in the urine (haematuria). Once local invasion has happened, and the basement membrane is breached, the tumour may come across lymphatic or blood vessels and be taken away on the flowing lymph or blood.

LYMPHATIC SPREAD

The lymphatic system comprises a series of vessels which convey a watery-based fluid, called lymph, back to the heart. The main role of the lymphatic system is to eliminate waste and cellular debris along with bacteria and proteins. When the cells of the body do their work, they produce waste which is discarded into the tissue space. As blood vessels become capillaries, plasma is pushed into this tissue space and this mixture of cellular debris, waste, proteins and maybe bacteria are taken up by the lymphatic vessels and transported away from that area. This important fact, that lymph is taken 'away' from an area (not to it), allows us to understand where a cancer is likely to spread.

As the lymph flows away, it comes across lymph nodes. There are many lymph nodes throughout the body, as seen in Fig. 1.15. A lymph node is a bean-shaped structure with a tough capsule round the outside. Inside is a fine meshwork of fibres designed to 'trap' any debris, proteins or bacteria. Inside this 'trap' are housed lymphocytes, white blood cells which are then programmed to destroy whatever needs destroying.

The cancer cell may be transported in flowing lymph and may become 'trapped' in a lymph node. Often, however, lymphocytes do not recognise the cancer cell and allow it to grow and replicate. Eventually, this group of malignant cells, along with an inflammatory response, will cause the node to swell. The patient may now experience an enlarged lymph node.

The drainage of lymph occurs in a very orderly way. It can be mapped out like roads are mapped out. If the lymph wants to flow from lymph node group A to lymph node group C, it will always go via B. This is referred to as 'contiguous' and demonstrates the orderly nature of lymph flow. Hodgkin lymphoma is a malignant neoplasm that involves the lymphatic system and vessels, and indeed it spreads from lymph node group to lymph node group in this contiguous fashion. 'Regional' lymphatic drainage can be defined as the first group(s) of lymph nodes that receive lymph from a particular area. The regional lymph nodes for areas of the body are very clearly defined in the tumour, node, metastasis (TNM) staging books, and involvement of these lymph nodes constitutes the 'N' category. For those involved in cancer registration, lymph node involvement outside of these designated nodes, referred to as 'extra-regional' would fall into the 'M' category of the TNM staging system.

Having identified the regional lymphatic drainage, these are the areas to be investigated first when a patient has a malignant tumour in a particular area. Most of the lymphatic drainage of the breast, for example, drains to the axillary lymph nodes, so this is the first place to investigate possible lymphatic involvement when a person has breast cancer.

The orderly nature of lymphatic flow makes lymphatic spread reasonably easy to understand and relatively easy to rule in or out. Spread via the blood, however, is not as orderly and is less easy to understand.

BLOOD SPREAD

Whereas the spread of cancer cells via the lymphatic system may seem quite logical and systematic and relatively easy to rule in or out, the same cannot be said with spread via the blood system. In the same way that local invasion can lead to lymphatic involvement, the cancer can also begin to invade blood vessels. Malignant cells may begin to grow along the inside of the blood vessel and this is called 'vascular invasion'. Cancer cells may break away from the tumour mass and be taken away on the flowing blood, just like a leaf on a river and which goes wherever the water goes; the same can be said for a cancer cell, which is tiny compared to the fast-flowing blood.

Cancer cells, in theory, can metastasise to anywhere within the body. However, they spread more readily to specific areas, and why this happens is not clearly understood. For example, when a breast cancer metastasises, it tends to metastasise to the brain and bone, prostate cancer tends to metastasise to the bones and when lung cancer metastasises, it tends to metastasise to the brain. This is known, because for many years patients with those primaries have returned with secondaries in these areas of the body. There are certain things that can be understood. For example, the normal blood flow from the intestines (small and large bowel) travels back to the heart via the liver. Therefore it is not unusual for a person with colon cancer to develop liver metastases. This is like a 'sow and seed' approach and is easier to understand. But why cancer spreads to other, seemingly more favourable parts of the body is more difficult to explain.

As stated earlier, metastases can develop anywhere in the body, but the four main areas tend to be the brain, bone, liver and lungs. Taking the lungs out of this equation, as there are as many primary lung tumours as secondary, primary tumours of the brain, liver and bone are extremely rare. It is more common to get secondaries in these areas than primaries.

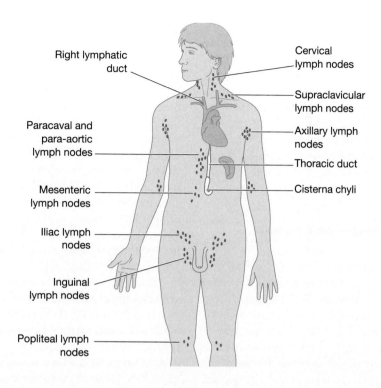

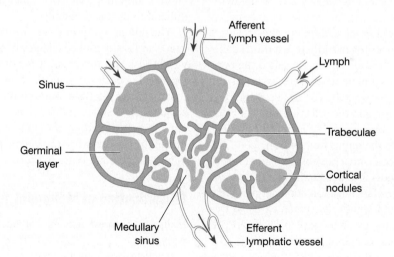

Fig. 1.15 The lymphatic system and lymph node.

That said, a tumour within, for example, the liver could still be a primary. The question remains, is it a secondary or a primary? Generally, when looking at malignant cells under a microscope, those cells still retain some characteristics of the 'parent' tissue. That is the tissue within which they are situated. So, with a primary of the liver, the cells of that primary would 'look' like liver cells (hepatocytes). However, if the tumour is a 'secondary', or metastasis, the cells of the metastasis would retain some of the characteristics of the tissue from where they originated (recall the earlier discuss about EMT and its reversal via MET). Those working within cancer registration will have noted that the morphology code for a metastasis is the same morphology code as the primary. This demonstrates that the cells originate from the same place (only the behaviour code changes: /6 vs /3). Metastases are tumours 'in' somewhere, not 'of' that somewhere. For example, a brain metastasis from a breast tumour is a breast tumour in the brain, not a tumour of the brain.

TRANSCOELOMIC SPREAD – ACROSS A BODY CAVITY

There are two body cavities of interest here, the thoracic cavity (chest) and the abdominopelvic cavity (abdomen and pelvis). These cavities are lined by a serous membrane, a membrane which consists of two layers; one (the parietal layer) attaches to the wall of the cavity, whilst the other (visceral layer) attaches to the organs within the cavity. In between the two membranes is fluid, called serum. This fluid is there to aid friction-free movement of the organs within the cavity.

In the thoracic cavity, the serous membrane is called the pleura, and in the abdominopelvic cavity, it is referred to as the peritoneum (there is a third serous membrane which surrounds the heart called the pericardium, but that is unimportant here as far as the spread of cancer is concerned). The serous membrane is an enclosed system, and the cells (mesothelial cells) making up the membranes are responsible for producing and reabsorbing the serous fluid within.

If the body is faced with a possible infection, one of its immediate defences is to produce fluid. This means that in the presence of an infection, for example, there is a build-up of fluid within the serous cavity. If this happens in the pleura it is called a 'pleural effusion'. If it happens in the peritoneum it is called 'ascites'.

A cancer involving these areas can produce a similar effect. A malignant neoplasm that affects the pleura is called 'mesothelioma' – note the cells lining these membranes are mesothelial cells; hence the name. Mesothelioma cells can float around the fluid to different parts of the lungs and begin to invade into the surface of the lungs, resulting in mesothelioma being problematic to cure, as it tends to involve the whole circumference of the lungs as a result of this transcoelomic spread.

Another area where this type of spread causes a problem is ovarian cancer. The ovaries sit within the peritoneum (partly) within the serous fluid, and if a cancer of the ovary breaks through its capsule, the malignant cells can float through the peritoneal fluid, maybe to the bottom of the pelvis. The body will recognise that these cells should not be there and as a defence will begin to secrete more serous fluid, more than can be reabsorbed, so there is a build-up of fluid. This means that there is more fluid for more cancer cells to float around, so the body tries to wash those away with more fluid, but this just means that there is more fluid for these can cells to float around, so the body produces more fluid.

This positive feedback loop results in the cancer cells floating around the abdominopelvic cavity and attach to the surface of the organs and structures that are found in this cavity. As a result, many women with ovarian cancer will experience 'malignant ascites', a build-up of fluid which has evidence of malignant cells. This results in malignant disease throughout the entire abdominopelvic cavity, and it is therefore very difficult to treat successfully.

The initial symptoms of ovarian cancer can be vague and easily missed: vague abdominal discomfort, weight loss and tiredness. It is not until the abdominal swelling occurs, the result of the malignant ascites, that diagnosis happens, but unfortunately that is often at quite a late stage. Transcoelomic spread from ovarian cancer throughout the abdominopelvic cavity is one of the reasons why survival for ovarian cancer lags behind some other types of cancer.

Classification of Malignant Tumours

Malignant tumours can be classified in a number of ways:

- Histopathological
- Location
- Biological
- Grade and stage

HISTOPATHOLOGICAL

Tumours can be classified according to their tissue of origin (Table 1.6).

TABLE 1.6   Tumour Terminology Related to Their Tissue of Origin

Tissue	Benign	Malignant
Epithelium	Papilloma	Carcinoma: basal cell carcinoma, squamous cell carcinoma, transitional cell carcinoma
Secretory or glandular epithelium	Adenoma	Adenocarcinoma
Connective		Sarcoma
Bone	Osteoma	Osteosarcoma
Cartilage	Chondroma	Chondrosarcoma
Fat	Lipoma	Liposarcoma
Fibrous	Fibroma	Fibrosarcoma
Voluntary muscles	Rhabdomyoma	Rhabdomyosarcoma
Involuntary muscles	Leiomyoma	Leiomyosarcoma
Tissue from foetal life		Blastoma

- Tumours that develop from epithelial cells, which are found in the linings of the skin, organs, digestive tract and airways, are termed carcinomas. This is the most common cancer type, accounting for approximately 80% to 90% of all cancers.
- Tumours arising from connective tissues such as muscle, bone, cartilage and fat are termed sarcomas.
- Childhood tumours often occur if embryonic/foetal tissue is left behind. These tumours are named after the blastocyte from which cells and tissues are derived in the embryo, such as nephroblastoma and neuroblastoma.
- Sometimes the tissue of origin cannot be determined because the cells are undifferentiated tumours. These tumours are classified as primary of unknown origin (PUO) or cancer of unknown primary (CUP) or simply unknown primary.

LOCATION

Often, a type of cancer will be categorised by its location; for example, cancer of the breast and cancer of the prostate. The actual site of any tumour is important in terms of symptoms, possible spread, treatment options and even prognosis. Treatment options will be different for a malignant melanoma of the retina compared with a malignant melanoma of the forearm. Also, a small tumour in the peripheral part of the lung may be treated differently from a tumour in the main bronchus.

BIOLOGICAL

Such a classification includes descriptions of the behaviour of the tumour, such as:

- Degree of differentiation (well, moderately, poorly, anaplastic)
  - As described earlier, the degree of differentiation (the grade) of a tumour is closely related to the potential metastasis. The more poorly differentiated the tumour is described as being, the greater the likelihood of metastasis. This is information that needs to be known at the outset of any patient management as it will help determine the most effective course of action.
- Lymphocyte positivity
  - Lymphocytes are a type of white blood cell that become active in response to a pathogen. They are an important part of the body's immune response. Tumours with infiltrating lymphocytes are recognised by the body, which then sets up an immune response. This lymphocyte positivity is often associated with increased response rates and better prognosis for cancer patients. Indeed, tumour-invading lymphocytes are being harvested and researched to form the basis of a newer, immunotherapeutic approach to cancer treatment.
- Hormone receptor status
  - Some tumours actively need hormones to survive. A woman's breast cancer might be referred to as oestrogen positive (*ER*+ve) Drugs such as tamoxifen and anastrozole (Arimidex) are designed to inhibit the uptake of oestrogen by the breast cancer cell, either by blocking

the receptor, in the case of tamoxifen, or by inhibiting the conversion of androgens by aromatase in post-menopausal women, as is the case with anastrozole. Both drugs are designed to interfere with the uptake of oestrogen by the cancer cell thereby inhibiting its growth potential.

- Oncogene status
  - As described earlier, cells are constantly receiving feedback and messages from their external environment, which stimulates the cells to grow and divide. Such messaging systems are known to be defective, and permanently active, in most cancer cells. A knowledge of which messaging system is involved and identification of the oncogenes within that process that are abnormal are leading the development of targeted drugs that can block the action of these proteins. One oncogene (a receptor on the cell surface) of particular note is the epidermal growth factor receptor (EGFR). EGFR has been shown to be mutated in 90% of squamous cell carcinomas of the head and neck and 80% of colorectal cancers; it is also commonly mutated in many lung cancers. Such knowledge is helping to personalise care for those with cancer that expresses such mutations.

TUMOUR GRADE

The classifications described above create an assessment of the tumour which affects the management options and prognosis of the patient. Tumours can also be categorised according to their grade and stage. Because all tumours are derived from a single rogue cell, it may be assumed that all subsequent cells should be identical or monoclonal; however, as the tumour cells continue to go through further cell cycles, they continue mutating so that a range of differentiations may be present within a tumour. The proportion of undifferentiated cells defines the grade of the tumour and provides an estimate of the degree of malignancy.

Generally, the grade is described on a scale of 1–4, as in Table 1.7. Sometimes a tumour can be so markedly undifferentiated that it is difficult to ascertain the tissue of origin. These are referred to as anaplastic tumours and are generally highly malignant, offering the worst prognosis.

TABLE 1.7 The Relationship Between Tumour Grade and Prognosis

Grade	Description	Prognosis
1	<25% undifferentiated cells	Better
2	>25%, <50% undifferentiated	↓
3	>50%, <75% undifferentiated	↓
4	>75% undifferentiated	Worse

For some tumour sites, it is necessary that a more accurate depiction of grade be assessed. An accurate assessment of grade in prostate cancer – the Gleason scale – is essential in determining the treatment and possible outcome for men with this disease. All grading scales essentially obey the underlying principles of grading; that is, how many cells look 'normal' (well differentiated) versus how many cells look 'abnormal' (poorly differentiated).

STAGING

Staging is a way in which the characteristics of cancer can be described. It allows clinicians to relate individual cases to the human body. It can therefore be referred to as an anatomical classification of the disease which helps to measure the size and extent of the tumour at the time of diagnosis. The uses of staging can be summarised as follows:

- Staging allows decisions to be made about the management of the cancer patient and helps to identify appropriate treatment(s).
- It allows similar cases to be compared, thus becoming a factor in estimating the prognosis of a case.
- It can aid in the development and evaluation of clinical trials, thereby allowing more effective management strategies to be developed.

TNM staging system developed jointly by the Union for International Cancer Control and the American Joint Committee on Cancer is widely recognised around the world as the principal staging system for most types of cancer. TNM forms the basis for cancer data collection within the UK as part of the National

Cancer Dataset and within US treatment facilities under the standards of the Commission on Cancer of the American College of Surgeons. Historically, there were many ways of staging different tumours, mainly dependent on the site within the body, which may lead to some confusion. Table 1.8 lists some of the other staging systems that are still used for certain primary cancers.

TNM staging describes the anatomic extent of the tumour; that is, how localised or how far spread the tumour is. It does this based on the assessment of three components:

- T – Extent of primary tumour
- N – Absence or presence and extent of regional lymph node involvement by the tumour
- M – Absence or presence of tumour at a distance from the primary site

By assigning numbers to these components (typically 0–4), an indication of the extent or severity of the disease can be made.

The T component represents the primary tumour and its size or extent at the site of origin. It can be classified according to the following general criteria:

- TX – Minimum requirements to assess the primary tumour cannot be met
- T0 – No evidence of primary tumour
- Tis – Carcinoma in situ
- T1– T4 – Progressive increase in tumour size and/or involvement of other structures

The definition of the T classification is relevant only for a particular tumour site and will vary. However, there are only two main ways in which tumour extension can be described: depth of invasion and size of tumour.

TABLE 1.8 **Some Staging Systems Other Than the Tumour-Node-Metastasis**	
Name of Staging Classification System	**Tumours**
Ann Arbor	Lymphomas (Hodgkin and non-Hodgkin)
The International Federation of Gynecology and Obstetrics (FIGO)	Gynaecological cancers: ovary, vagina and endometrial cervix
Dukes	Colorectal cancers

Depth of invasion tends to be used when the tumour site is in a 'hollow' organ (Fig. 1.16A), such as in the bladder, oesophagus or colon, where the organ typically has a lumen surrounded by layers of tissue; for example, mucosa, submucosa, muscularis and serosa.

The size of the tumour tends to be used when the tumour site is in a parenchymal (solid) organ (see Fig. 1.16B). Parenchymal organs, such as the liver, breast and lungs, have a specific function. Here, tumours will be described as 2 cm in the greatest diameter, for example.

The N component describes regional lymph node involvement and can be categorised according to the following:

- Nx – Minimum requirements to assess the regional lymph nodes cannot be met.
- N0 – No evidence of regional lymph node involvement.
- N1 – N3 – Increasing involvement of regional lymph nodes in size, number, location or other factors.

It is important to note that the N category only applies to regional lymph nodes that are specifically listed in the TNM staging manual. Involvement of other distant nodes is classified in the M category.

The M category also describes the spread of the tumour via the blood to distant sites of the body.

- M0 – No evidence of distant metastases
- M1 – Presence of distant metastases

Additional notations may be added to highlight the site of the metastases, such as pulmonary (PUL), liver (HEP) and brain (BRA).

Each of these categories can be further annotated with a lowercase 'c' or 'p'. These refer to a clinical (c) stage and a pathological or post-surgical (p) stage.

CLINICAL STAGE (c) – cTNM OR TNM

A clinical stage is given based on evidence that can be seen through initial investigations. For example, a clinician may find a 2-cm tumour on a computed tomography (CT) scan of a patient with a suspected lung cancer. The same scan may also reveal evidence of enlarged lymph nodes. Based on these clinical findings, this case can be given a (clinical) stage. Note here that the 'c' is mostly absent.

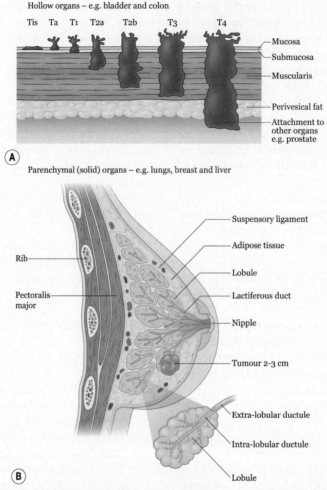

Fig. 1.16 T stage. (A) Hollow organs – e.g. bladder and colon. (B) Parenchymal (solid) organs – e.g. lungs, breast and liver.

The clinical stage would suggest that lung cancer is present, and surgery is needed to remove the tumour. The resection would be sent to the pathology laboratory for further investigation by the pathologist.

PATHOLOGICAL (POST-SURGICAL) STAGE (P) – PTNM

Further investigation by the pathologist might reveal that the tumour is in fact 5 cm and more lymph nodes are involved than was originally indicated. From this further analysis, the case is upstaged and the notation 'p' is used to describe this. The 'p' stage indicates that further (adjunct) treatment is required.

Cancer registries throughout the world may also be aware of a third stage called the integrated stage, where a combination of the clinical and pathological stages is used to best represent the overall stage for this case.

Once the T, N and M categories have been noted, they are grouped to give a stage. Excluding the X category, there are 48 different permutations of these components: T (0–4, is), N (0–3) and M (0–1). These permutations are assigned to broader categories called stage groups to give an indication of the likely prognosis and treatment strategy. Table 1.9 shows the stage grouping definitions for TNM.

TABLE 1.9   Stage Group Definitions

Stage Classification	Stage Group
Carcinoma in situ	0
Tumours localised to organ of origin	I & II
Locally extensive spread, particularly to local lymph nodes	III
Distant metastasis	IV

The classification of cancer, along with the stage and grade, forms the basis of an overall plan of treatment for a specific case. Such a treatment may use a combination of methods. The three main treatment strategies for cancer are surgery, radiotherapy and chemotherapy. Other therapies such as immunotherapy, hormone therapy and biological therapies also play an important role in the treatment of cancer.

Treatment of Cancer

To be effective against cancer, a treatment plan must take into consideration the stage and grade of the disease. If detected at an early stage, the disease may be dealt with using a local treatment such as surgery, whereas if it is not identified until at a later stage, when the disease has metastasised, a more systemic approach to treatment is required, such as chemotherapy. Likewise, patients deemed to have high-grade tumours may be offered chemotherapy, as the chance of metastasis is high, whereas patients with low-grade tumours have a low risk of metastasis.

SURGERY

Surgery plays an important role in both the treatment of cancer and in diagnosis and staging. It is a local treatment designed to remove all or part of the tumour at the primary site. Diagnostic samples (biopsies) can be removed and sent for further analysis to allow a histopathological diagnosis to be made. At the time of surgery, the surgeon may also take a sample from the lymph nodes to see if they have any involvement, thereby providing information for the N classification. The extent of the primary within the organ or tissue (T) can similarly be established.

Surgery, as a treatment modality, is able to control the primary tumour. It is also essential to recognise that many cancers may recur at the site of origin, making wide excision essential in some cases. Recognition of the role of other therapies such as radiotherapy has, however, led to a more conservative approach to some surgical techniques. For example, in the early to mid-1900s, breast cancer was traditionally treated using a radical or total mastectomy. Clinical trials in the 1970s and 1980s demonstrated that this may not always be necessary and that local excision of the tumour followed by radiotherapy to the breast could offer as good a chance of cure while keeping the breast intact.

RADIOTHERAPY

Radiotherapy is the treatment of cancer using high-energy ionising radiation. Ionising radiation is harmful to living tissue and, as such, it is necessary to control exposure to it. Again, it is predominantly a localised treatment, which can be broadly divided into two groups: external beam radiotherapy and brachytherapy.

External beam radiotherapy uses radiation that is created electronically by a linear accelerator, often referred to as a LINAC. Directed from a source outside the patient, the radiation aims to traverse the patient and deposit its energy in the tissue and tumour.

The deposition of energy inside the cell leads to the formation of free radicals, which are highly reactive agents that cause damage within the cell. Such damage (single- and double-strand DNA breaks) subsequently causes the cell to die.

The killing of cells with radiation is largely non-discriminatory. The radiation kills healthy cells as well as tumour cells, so care must be taken to ensure that little damage is received from normal healthy tissue. Careful planning is required to direct the radiation to the 'tumour volume', while at the same time making sure that the radiation dose is minimised so that it does not affect potential 'organs at risk'.

It is known that normal, otherwise healthy cells repair and recover from radiation damage better than an abnormal, mutated, tumour cell. This is the main reason why radiotherapy tends to be given in 'fractions' (a daily dose) over many days.

Fig. 1.17 demonstrates how fractionation can be used to incrementally kill more tumour cells. Starting with 100% of cells (both healthy and tumourous), the first fraction (dose of radiation) is delivered. As radiation kills cells, it can be expected that the lines will fall as cells die off. Notice how the normal cells die off at the same rate as the tumour cell – radiation will kill them both equally as well!

However, notice also that after waiting 24 hours the lines begin to rise. This is a result of normal and tumour cells recovering from the radiation damage, but the tumour line has not recovered quite as well as the normal cell line. When the next fraction is delivered, the lines drop again. The following process is repeated: fraction, drop, recover, fraction, drop, recover. And over the 25 or 30 fractions of radiotherapy, we will begin to see a difference in the rates of cell death.

It is important to note that the normal cell line is still falling, just not quite as much. Thus, damage to normal tissue is still experienced and side effects will result. These include epilation (local hair loss), erythema (reddening of the skin like sunburn) and mucositis (inflammation of the mucous membrane; for example, in the mouth).

Brachytherapy (*brachys* = Greek for 'short range') is a medical treatment that involves the placement of small radioactive sources within a natural body cavity, through tissue or close to the surface. It is unlike the linear accelerator, where the radiation source disappears as soon as the device is switched off. Indeed, the physics behind brachytherapy means that the radiation is deposited in a short range of tissue, allowing high doses to be given to the tumour without necessarily irradiating too much healthy tissue. Brachytherapy can be administered in a variety of ways:

- Intracavity – the radioactive sources are placed into a cavity within the body; for example, the uterus.
- Intraluminal – the radioactive sources are placed into a lumen of the body; for example, the oesophagus.
- Interstitial – the radioactive sources are placed through tissue; for example, implants for prostate cancer.

CHEMOTHERAPY

Chemotherapy refers to the use of drugs to combat the disease process. More accurately, it should be referred to as cytotoxic chemotherapy because the drugs used

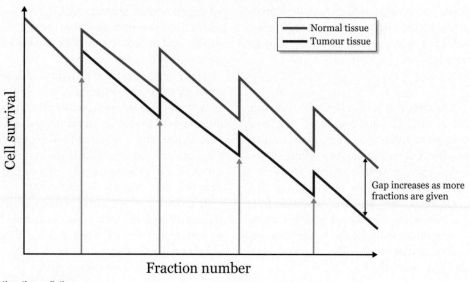

Fractionating radiotherapy

Cell survival

Fraction number

Fig. 1.17 Fractionating radiotherapy.

to fight the cancer have a cytotoxic (cell-killing) effect. Chemotherapy drugs work by halting or disrupting the normal cell cycle (see Fig. 1.3).

Different categories of chemotherapy drugs work in different ways but, essentially, they stop DNA from forming or somehow interact directly with it. Either way, the cell fails to replicate and therefore dies.

ANTI-METABOLITES

This category of drugs relies on the fact that the cell needs certain components to be able to function and replicate DNA. These can be divided into purine (adenine and guanine) analogues, pyrimidine (thymine and cytosine [uracil in RNA]) analogues and anti-folates.

Purines and pyrimidines are the essential building blocks of DNA, referred to as 'bases'. DNA is made up of a complex series of these bases, which are ordered in a certain way. A segment of the DNA containing these bases provides the instructions for producing proteins within the cell. Without these four bases – adenine, thymine, cytosine and guanine – DNA cannot replicate properly and the cell will die.

Anti-metabolite chemotherapy drugs prevent these substances from being incorporated into the DNA, thereby stopping cell replication.

Anti-folates are another group of drugs within this category. Folinic acid is required by the cell to allow the production of purines and pyrimidines. As seen above, these are the essential components of DNA. Anti-folates work by impairing the function and production of folinic acid, thereby halting the production of purines and pyrimidines, which in turn stops cell replication and leads to cell death. Methotrexate is one example of an anti-metabolite chemotherapy drug that is used for a wide range of cancers. See Table 1.10 for further examples of drugs within this category.

ALKYLATING AGENTS

The nitrogenous bases of DNA join in a particular way. Adenine will only join onto thymine, while guanine will only join onto cytosine. Alkylating agent chemotherapy works by directly targeting the DNA and causing bonds across bases where there should not be one. They are designed to produce covalent bonds between guanine bases. Such bonds will interfere with DNA replication and the cell will die.

TABLE 1.10 Examples of Anti-Metabolite Chemotherapy Drugs (not exhaustive)

Purine Analogues	Pyrimidine Analogues	Antifolates
• Mercaptopurine • Thioguanine (used to treat acute leukaemias) • Fludarabine • Pentostatin and cladribine (adenosine analogues that are used primarily to treat hairy cell leukaemia)	• 5-Fluorouracil (inhibits thymidylate synthase) • Cytosine arabinoside (cytarabine, Ara-C) • Gemcitabine	• Methotrexate • Pemetrexed

Because this form of chemotherapy directly targets the DNA, it is possible that the damaged cell will try to repair itself or still replicate but in a damaged format. This is not ideal and may even lead to cancer, as alkylating agents are known carcinogens. For example, those who work in the coding world may be aware of a code in the *International Classification of Diseases* diagnostics tool for therapy-related acute myeloid leukaemia with a sub-bullet point for alkylating agent chemotherapy. It is possible for people to return with a second form of cancer possibly caused by the drugs given to them to cure them of an initial cancer.

Platinum-based drugs such as carboplatin and others are considered alkylating-like as they also cause bonds; however, they do not use an 'alkyl' group to cause the bond but instead use a molecule of platinum to cause the bond between the guanine bases. The net result is the same – the cell struggles to replicate properly and dies.

Examples of alkylating agent chemotherapy drugs can be seen in Table 1.11.

TOPOISOMERASE INHIBITORS

DNA is immensely long and needs to be tightly coiled and wound up to fit into the tiny nucleus. Therefore for the DNA to be able to replicate it needs to uncoil. An enzyme called topoisomerase (pronounced topoisom erase) allows this to happen. Indeed, without this enzyme to help uncoil DNA in an orderly fashion,

TABLE 1.11 Alkylating Agent Chemotherapy (Not Exhaustive)	
Alkylating Agent	**Alkylating-Like**
• Cyclophosphamide • Mechlorethamine or mustine (HN2) (trade name Mustardgen) • Uramustine or uracil mustard • Melphalan • Chlorambucil • Ifosfamide • Carmustine • Lomustine • Streptozocin • Busulfan	• Cisplatin • Carboplatin • Oxaliplatin • Satraplatin

the DNA cannot splice apart easily and the cell will die. There are two types of topoisomerase inhibitors, and these are designed to stop the DNA unwinding: topoisomerase I (topotecan, irinotecan) and topoisomerase II (etoposide, teniposide) inhibitors. Topoisomerase II inhibitors are also known carcinogens and, in a small number of cases, have put patients at risk of acquiring acute myeloid leukaemia 2 to 3 years after initial treatment.

ANTI-TUMOUR ANTIBIOTICS

Common among these types of agents is their interference with cell division. Some are derived from bacteria and produce powerful free radicals, which damage the DNA of the cell and cause cell death.

The anthracyclines are a particularly notable class of anti-tumour antibiotics, which include drugs such as doxorubicin, adriamycin, idarubicin and epirubicin. Such drugs are known to cause damage to the heart and often come with a lifetime dose limit. Patients receiving these drugs are assessed and monitored for heart problems before and after receiving treatment.

Other (non-anthracycline) drugs in this category would include bleomycin, mitomycin and actinomycin.

MITOTIC INHIBITORS

When a cell is ready to divide, it enters the mitosis phase of the cell cycle. As the cell begins to cleave apart, the two new cells are momentarily joined by the formation of microtubules. Once the cell is completely satisfied that division can occur, the microtubules are disassembled, and two separated cells result. Two groups of mitotic inhibitor drugs prevent this cell division from occurring: vinca alkaloids and taxanes. But their mechanism of action is juxtaposed.

VINCA ALKALOIDS

Originally harvested and derived from the Periwinkle plant, vinca alkaloids bind to tubulin and thereby prevent assembly of the microtubules. The original vinca alkaloids include vincristine and vinblastine. Other semi-synthetic drugs now exist such as vinorelbine, vindesine and vinflunine.

TAXANES

These drugs were also harvested from natural sources. The first, paclitaxel, was derived from the Pacific yew tree. Now, paclitaxel (as well as another taxane called docetaxel) is produced semi-synthetically. In contrast to vinca alkaloids, these drugs promote microtubule stability, which prevents their disassembly. The net result is the same: the cell cannot cleave apart and will therefore die.

Like radiotherapy, chemotherapy is given in discrete bouts of treatment, referred to as cycles. A full cycle of chemotherapy comprises the time taken to give the drugs along with a rest period for the patient. Within a typical cycle length of 21 days, the drugs tend to be administered between days 1 and 5 (D1–5). The patient will then have 16 days' rest before receiving the next dose of chemotherapy. The second cycle starts again at D1.

Cycles of chemotherapy work on the same basis as radiotherapy fractionation. The rest period allows the human body to recover just enough to tolerate the next dose of chemotherapy. Although this time also allows tumour tissue to recover, as mentioned previously, normal cells recover better than tumour cells. Once again, this differential can be accentuated over a number of cycles.

Also, like radiotherapy, chemotherapy drugs are non-discriminatory; that is, they affect healthy as well as tumour cells and therefore side effects can occur (Table 1.12). Generally, the more frequently a cell divides, the more sensitive it is to the chemotherapy drug, which is why noted side effects tend to occur in

TABLE 1.12 Common Side Effects of Chemotherapy	
General	**Organ Specific and Other**
• Bone marrow suppression • Hair loss – alopecia • Nausea and vomiting • Appetite and weight loss • Taste changes • Sores in mouth and throat • Fatigue	• Heart damage (cardiac toxicity) – daunorubicin and doxorubicin • Nervous system changes (peripheral nerves) – mitotic inhibitors such as vincristine • Lung damage (pneumotoxicity) – bleomycin • Liver and kidney damage • Long-term side effects • Secondary cancers

those areas of the body with fast-dividing tissue, such as in mucous membranes, the digestive tract and bone marrow.

BIOLOGICAL (TARGETED) THERAPY

Radiotherapy and chemotherapy are powerful treatment strategies designed to kill tumour cells effectively. However, they also do too much damage to the healthy tissue and patient. Indeed, many people are employed in hospitals and clinics to deal with the after effects of the treatments rather than the cancer itself.

This is partly because radiotherapy and chemotherapy do not really pay attention to the differences between healthy cells and tumour cells. A difference is manufactured in radiotherapy by using different angled beams, conformal and intensity-modulated radiotherapy, as well as fractionation. With regard to chemotherapy, patients with cancer sometimes receive a combination of drugs that have different modes of action and side effects. By using these strategies, an incrementally greater effect of radiotherapy and chemotherapy on tumours over healthy cells can be manufactured.

In contrast, biological therapies consider the difference between tumour cells and normal cells. All cells rely on a signalling pathway that converts messages (which usually come from outside the cell) to actions: the cell will grow, it will divide, it may move and it may die. In cancer, this signalling pathway is disrupted by damage and mutation, which can lead to aberrant and incorrect messages being received. Herein lie the differences between tumour cells and normal cells. What exactly are these differences?

Fig. 1.18 demonstrates how a cancer cell can be distinguished from a normal cell, and Table 1.13 shows how these differences can be further divided into targets that appear on the outside of the cell (extracellular) and those that appear on the inside of the cell (intracellular).

EXTRACELLULAR TARGETS

All cells rely on messages being received and interpreted. Cancer cells produce many messages (ligands, growth factors) which will influence other cancer cells around them to grow and proliferate. As described earlier, a tumour only has to grow a few millimetres in diameter before it needs more oxygen, which it will derive from creating a new blood supply (angiogenesis).

A powerful stimulant of angiogenesis is VEGF. Tumour cells will secrete vast quantities of VEGF, which will interact with nearby blood vessels, instructing them to send tributaries to the tumour.

New angiogenesis inhibitor drugs, such as bevacizumab (Avastin) and sorafenib inhibit the attachment of VEGF onto the endothelial (cells lining the blood vessel walls), thereby stopping the message to produce a new blood vessel.

Such an approach is designed to prevent blood vessel formation in and around the tumour, starving it of oxygen and nutrients and limiting a potential route for metastasis. Unfortunately, blood vessel formation is also important in many normal body processes, such as wound healing, heart and kidney function, foetal development and reproduction. Side effects of treatment with angiogenesis inhibitors can include problems with bleeding, clots in the arteries (with resultant stroke or heart attack), hypertension and protein in the urine.

OVERACTIVE RECEPTOR AND OVEREXPRESSION OF RECEPTOR

In some cancers, a cell surface receptor can be overactive, meaning it is permanently in the 'on' state and transmitting messages to the cell even in the absence of a growth factor. The epidermal growth factor receptor (EGFR) is known to be overactive in many colorectal cancers and squamous cell carcinomas of the head and

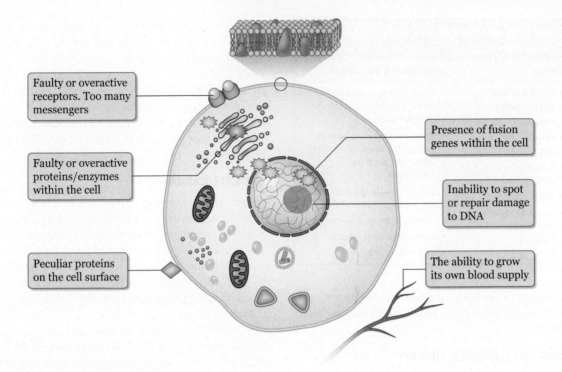

Faulty or overactive receptors. Too many messengers

Faulty or overactive proteins/enzymes within the cell

Peculiar proteins on the cell surface

Presence of fusion genes within the cell

Inability to spot or repair damage to DNA

The ability to grow its own blood supply

Fig. 1.18 What makes a cancer cell different?

TABLE 1.13 Extracellular and Intracellular Differences of a Cancer Cell	
Extracellular Differences/ Targets	**Intracellular Differences/ Targets**
• Too many ligands (messengers) – epidermal growth factor; vascular endothelial growth factor • Overactive receptor – epidermal growth factor receptor • Overexpression of receptor – HER2 (breast cancer) • Peculiar proteins on cell surface – CD20, CD30, CD52	• Mutation in a signalling protein so that it is constitutively active – keeps telling cell to divide even in the absence of the message (BRAF, KRAS) • Mutation in the DNA machinery fusion genes (Philadelphia chromosome, ALK) • Tumour suppressor genes not working (p53, PTEN, Rb)

neck. Drugs such as cetuximab (Erbitux) and panitumumab (Vectibix) attach to the extracellular portion of EGFR and block the binding site for the growth factor (message). Small-molecule inhibitors, such as gefitinib, erlotinib, brigatinib and lapatinib, bind to the intracellular portion of EGFR. Such binding prevents EGFR from activation, which is a prerequisite for the binding of downstream adaptor proteins. This results in the halting of the signalling cascade in cells that rely on this pathway for growth, tumour proliferation and migration.

HER2 (neu, ERB2) is an example of a receptor that is often over-expressed on the surface of breast cancer cells. Damage to the genes of the cell may result in too many HER2 receptors being produced. As a result, the cell will naturally receive too many messages to divide, proliferate and potentially metastasise. Trastuzumab (Herceptin) attaches to HER2 and blocks its action. Pertuzumab (Perjeta) can also block its action but in a slightly different way.

PECULIAR, OR PARTICULAR, PROTEINS ON THE CELL SURFACE

Some cancers will express particular proteins on the surface of the cell that can be used as a target. For example, most follicular non-Hodgkin lymphomas will express CD20, which is the target for rituximab (Rituxan, MabThera). Rituximab works by attracting and improving the work of T cells in destroying these cells. Ofatumumab, ocrelizumab and obinutuzumab are examples of other drugs that target the CD20 proteins in cancer cells.

INTRACELLULAR TARGETS

It is possible to target the internal portion of an overactive receptor. As suggested above, small-molecule inhibitors such as gefitinib are designed to target the internal portion of EGFR in lung cancers that are EGFR+ve (about 10% to 15%).

MUTATION IN A SIGNALLING PROTEIN

It is known that with some cancers there can be damage, a mutation, in the proteins that transfer messages to the nucleus. These signalling proteins, including BRAF, KRAS and MEK, are known to be mutated in certain cancers, such that the signalling pathway is constitutively active, even in the absence of a ligand–receptor interaction. Half of malignant melanomas have BRAF mutations, and drugs like vemurafenib and

dabrafenib are designed to inhibit the action of this mutated protein.

MUTATION IN THE DNA MACHINERY

Such mutation can fall into two categories: the creation of fusion genes and the disruption of tumour suppressor genes such as P53, Rb and PTEN.

Genetic events, including gene translocations and deletions, can cause the formation of fusion genes, whereby two previously separate genes are rearranged to create a hybrid gene. The Philadelphia chromosome is one example of such a gene, and while it is generally associated with chronic myeloid leukaemia, it can also be seen in other types of leukaemia and lymphoma. The Philadelphia chromosome, or *BCR/ABL*, gene results when a portion of chromosome 22 and a portion of chromosome 9 swap over (Fig. 1.19). Such a swapping over of genetic material is called a 'translocation' in is represented as t(9:22); 9 and 22 represent the numbers of the chromosomes involved in the exchange.

The Philadelphia chromosome promotes white blood cell growth and replication; it is the driving force behind chronic myeloid leukaemia. Drugs such

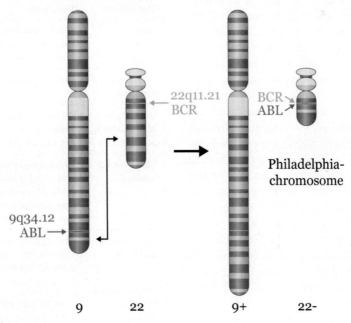

Fig. 1.19 The Philadelphia chromosome.

as imatinib, dasatinib, nilotinib and, more recently, radotinib and bosutinib are designed to combat the action of this fusion gene and halt the progress of the disease.

Tumour suppressor genes play an important role in preventing cancer from occurring in our cells. Such genes are responsible for monitoring whether damage occurs within the cell (DNA) and facilitating repair. If a repair cannot be achieved, then the tumour suppressor gene may initiate apoptosis (programmed cell death). These types of genes protect the cell from progressing on the path towards cancer. Therefore if they mutate, causing a loss or reduction in their function, the cell can then become cancerous. Other factors, as discussed earlier, are also required to enable cancer to fully develop, but tumour suppressor genes are crucial in this whole turn of events. Failure to develop treatment strategies to reinsert tumour suppressor genes, or to make them operative once again, means that targeting tumour suppressor genes with effective treatment has so far eluded scientists.

Biological (targeted) therapies use monoclonal antibodies (mAbs) and small-molecule inhibitors to target the mutated protein. mAbs are large structures (comparatively), and any target needs to be extracellular (on a surface or ligand). It also needs to be big enough for the mAb to bind to (such as a protein) and something that the cell needs to survive. If the mAb is designed to attract immune cells, as is the case with rituximab, then there need to be immune cells present in and around the tumour. Furthermore, any target needs to present, ideally, only on cancer cells or over-expressed.

Small-molecule inhibitors, on the other hand, are small enough to enter the cell membrane and interact (compete for) binding sites within the cell itself. As many of the binding sites within the signal cascade are similar, small-molecule inhibitors tend to be less specific and can possibly interact with several targets.

The term 'targeted' therapy therefore is a bit of a misnomer and needs further clarification. The presence of receptors and the use of the signal cascade is a process that is normal and common to all cells within the body. The fact that they are mutated (over-expressed) in cancer cells make them a useful target but not an exclusive one! The net result is that patients still experience side effects.

Many targeted therapy drugs cause a rash or other skin changes that can range from mild to severe. Skin problems occur because many of the drugs used target aberrant EGFR, which is mutated in many cancers and is a useful target. But EGFR is found naturally on many other cells within the body. For example, epithelial cells of the skin have many EGF receptors and, as such, are quickly damaged by drugs (e.g. cetuximab and erlotinib) that target this receptor in EGFR+ve disease.

Interestingly, it has been demonstrated that certain side effects may be associated with a better patient outcome. For example, patients who develop an acneiform rash (skin eruptions that resemble acne) while being treated with the inhibitors erlotinib or gefitinib have tended to respond better to these drugs than patients who do not develop the rash.

Table 1.14 lists some common and less common side effects of targeted treatments.

IMMUNOTHERAPY

Immunotherapy is the name given to treatments that initiate the body to fight against cancer. These

TABLE 1.14 Side Effects to Targeted Therapies	
Side Effects	**Comments**
Skin	More common with EGFR targeted therapy; can range from dry skin to severe acne, which is itchy and sore
High blood pressure	Anti-angiogenic drugs
Bleeding or blood clotting problems	Anti-angiogenic drugs can cause bruising and bleeding; internal bleeding can be life-threatening
Slow wound healing	Anti-angiogenic drugs can interfere with wound healing, such as old wounds opening and new wounds not closing; can also lead to perforations in the stomach or intestine
Autoimmune reactions	Checkpoint inhibitors (more detail on these later) may take the brakes off immune system, allowing it to attack the body's own cells and tissues
Other side effects	Nausea and vomiting; diarrhoea or constipation; mouth sores

types of drugs are sometimes referred to as biological response modifiers because they promote the body's own response to fight an infection (in this case cancer). Immunotherapy can be local – as in the treatment of carcinoma of the bladder, where BCG is administered directly into the bladder via a catheter – or it can be systemic, where the drug is used to treat the whole body, such as interferon or interleukin 2, which have been shown to be effective against kidney cancer. Moreover, immunotherapy drugs can be given to boost the body's natural defence system (termed non-specific immunotherapy) or they can be used to target individual tumour cells and not normal cells. Such an approach tends to use mAbs.

To appreciate how mAbs can be used in an immunotherapy approach to cancer treatment, it is first necessary to look at how the immune system works in relation to cancer. At the beginning of this book, the hallmarks of cancer were listed. Notice that in 2011 two further hallmarks were added, one of which was the tumour's ability to evade the body's immune system.

Immune cells (T cells) scan the body's other cells and tissues, searching for foreign bodies, bacteria, viruses and cancer cells. As the T cell approaches a normal body cell, there is an interaction in which the normal cell is 'seen' as normal by the T cell and left alone. The T cell probes for certain proteins that serve as identifying markers for healthy, normal cells. If the proteins indicate that the cell is infected or cancerous, the T cell will lead an attack against it.

Programmed cell death 1 (PD-1) and cytotoxic T-lymphocyte-associated antigen 4 (CTLA-4) are the probes that the T cell uses to seek out infected or cancerous cells. Programmed cell death ligand 1 (PD-L1) is the protein on the normal cell that interacts with PD-1 and indicates to the T cell to leave them alone. Such an interaction is called a checkpoint and is analogous to a 'molecular handshake', indicating that all is well. However, it appears that cancer cells are also good at producing proteins such as PD-L1. The result is that when a circulating T cell comes across a cancerous cell which expresses PD-L1, the molecular handshake takes place and fools the T cell into thinking the cancer cell is in fact a normal cell and can be left alone.

A range of drugs called checkpoint inhibitors can either block these normal proteins on cancer cells or the proteins on T cells that respond to them. Consequently, this removes the molecular handshake that prevents T cells from recognising the cells as cancerous and allows for an immune system assault on the cancer cells. Such checkpoint inhibitors – for example, ipilimumab (PD-1), pembrolizumab (PD-1) and nivolumab (CTLA-4) – block the molecular handshake by interacting directly with the T cell probe. Atezolizumab is another checkpoint inhibitor; however, this drug interacts with PD-L1 found on the antigen-presenting cell. Fig. 1.20 shows the interaction of these drugs with T cells and cancer cells.

These and other immune checkpoint therapies represent one of the most promising cancer treatment strategies to date, with encouraging results found in patients with advanced melanoma and lymphoma.

A word of caution, however. By releasing the brakes on the immune system, the molecular handshake for all cells can potentially be withdrawn. This is a crucial protective mechanism that stops T cells from attacking healthy, normal cells and, without it, normal body cells are potentially open to attack from their own immune system, which could cause catastrophic auto-immune-type responses. Common side effects include fatigue, cough, nausea, loss of appetite, skin rash and itching. More serious problems might be seen in the lungs, intestines, liver, kidneys, hormone-producing glands and other organs.

THE MULTIDISCIPLINARY APPROACH TO THE TREATMENT OF CANCER

Much has been done over the past decade to bring groups of professionals together to focus on benefitting individual patients with cancer. Such groups are called multidisciplinary teams. They comprise diverse disciplines that provide comprehensive assessment and consultation for a particular cancer case. While primarily there to help team members resolve difficult cases, teams may also fulfil a variety of additional functions. For example, they can help promote coordination between different professionals, provide a 'checks and balances' mechanism to ensure that the interests and rights of all concerned parties (particularly the patient) are addressed and perhaps identify service gaps and breakdowns in coordination or communication. They also enhance the professional skills and knowledge of individual team members by providing a forum for

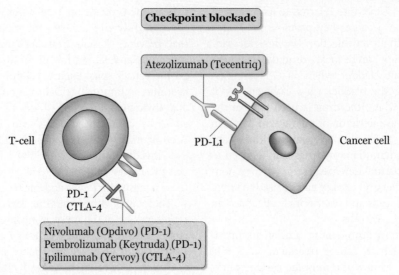

Fig. 1.20 Checkpoint inhibitors. *CTLA-4*, Cytotoxic T-lymphocyte associated antigen 4; *PD-1*, programmed cell death 1; *PD-L1*, programmed cell death ligand 1.

learning more about different strategies, resources and approaches used across various disciplines for cancer treatment. Such an approach to the treatment of individual cancer cases is essential for providing appropriate management strategies and attaining the best possible chance of cure for the patient.

SELF-ASSESSMENT QUESTIONS

Answer true or false to the following. Answers are on page 165–166.

1 *In situ suggests the carcinoma cells are breaching the basement membrane.*

2 *A well-differentiated tumour is one that is unlike its parent tissue.*

3 *A tumour developing from epithelial tissue is given the term sarcoma.*

4 *Staging refers to the level of differentiation of a neoplasm.*

5 *All cells that are capable of division are able to become malignant tumours.*

6 *The grade of a tumour refers to its size and extent.*

7 *A benign tumour grows by extension and invasion.*

8 *A benign tumour does not metastasise.*

9 *Cancer results from the controlled proliferation of body cells.*

10 *Malignant tumours will always have the potential to metastasise.*

11 *A benign tumour of fibrous tissue is called a fibroma.*

12 *Adenocarcinoma refers to tumours of adipose tissue.*

13 *Simple epithelial tissue has more than two layers.*

14 *Transitional epithelium has many layers so that it can expand.*

15 *The traditional staging system for gynaecological tumours is the Dukes' system.*

16 *Pleomorphism refers to the presence of normal-looking nuclei within cells.*

17 *Proto-oncogenes promote normal cells to grow and replicate.*

18 *The T classification in the TNM staging system involves the size/depth of the tumour.*

19 *A classification of M1 suggests late-stage disease.*

20 *Grade 1 would suggest also stage I.*

Blood Cancers

Chapter Outline

Objectives

By the end of this chapter the reader should be able to:

- Give an overview of the circulatory system.
- Relate the maturation of blood cells to the different types of blood cancer.
- Understand the similarities and differences between leukaemia, lymphoma and myeloma.
- Describe the classifications of leukaemia, lymphoma and myeloma.
- Relate the genetic variants of blood cancer to respective targeted treatments.
- Outline the likely treatment options available for patients with blood cancer.

The term circulatory system describes the cardiovascular and the lymphatic systems working together. Both consist of moving fluids necessary to transport essential minerals, proteins, gases and other substances throughout the body. The vessels of the cardiovascular system form a closed-circuit network that continually transports blood around the body. In contrast, lymphatic vessels begin as blind-ended vessels within tissue spaces. Lymph is ultimately conveyed back into the blood via a series of lymphatic vessels.

The Cardiovascular System

The cardiovascular system comprises the heart and blood vessels: namely, arteries, veins and capillaries (Fig. 2.1). The function of the heart is to pump blood around the body, and the blood is conveyed by arteries that generally take oxygenated blood away from the heart. Major arteries, such as the aorta, are responsible for the first part of this transportation. As the blood reaches organs or tissues where the oxygen is required, the arteries become ever smaller until ultimately they form capillaries that have walls one cell

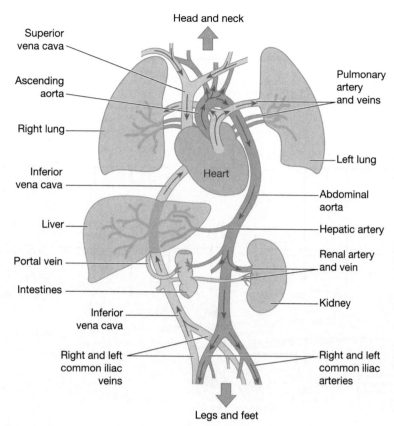

Fig. 2.1 The cardiovascular system.

layer thick to enable the exchange of gases between the blood and tissue. Oxygen is absorbed into the tissue in exchange for carbon dioxide. This new blood, now without oxygen, transports carbon dioxide and other waste materials back towards the heart via small veins (venules) that join together to form larger veins. The two largest veins in the body are the superior and inferior vena cava. The superior vena cava transports the blood from the head and neck area back towards the heart, and the inferior vena cava transports blood from the lower part of the body back to the heart.

BLOOD

Blood is made up of blood cells (45% – red, white and platelets) and plasma (55%). Plasma contains mainly water, proteins, gases, electrolytes, hormones and other materials. The main function of the blood is to transport essential goods to tissues of the body and to transport waste material away from those tissues and out of the body.

Haematopoiesis (blood cell formation) takes place in the red bone marrow located in various parts of the body. In adults, red bone marrow can be found in the epiphyses of the humerus and femur; a few irregular or flat bones such as the vertebra, pelvic bones and sternum; and some lymphatic tissues, such as the lymph nodes, spleen and thymus. The blood cells originate from pluripotential stem cells – that is, a single stem cell has the potential to differentiate (mature) into any of the types of blood cells. The differentiation pathway can be seen in Fig. 2.2. It is important to recognise that the pluripotential stem cell, found at the beginning of the pathway, may proceed down either of two paths: the myeloid cell path or the lymphoid cell path.

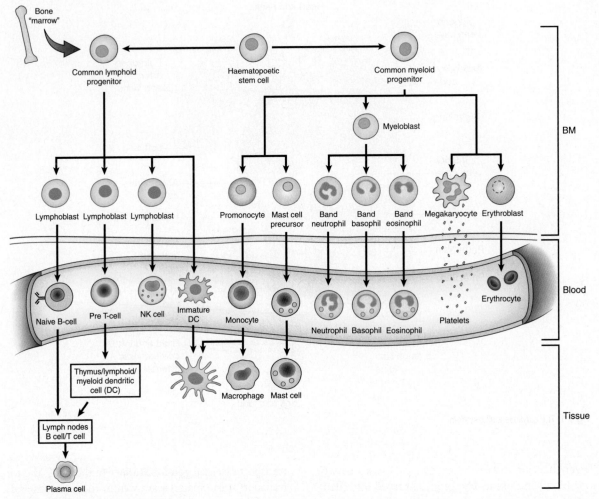

Fig. 2.2 Differentiation pathway of blood cells.

Each pathway will result in a variety of blood cells. The names of these cells and their functions can be found in Table 2.1. White cells, which can be further subdivided into granulocytes (those cells with granules in the cytoplasm) and agranulocytes (those without granules), play a major role in the body's immune response.

It is important to understand the pathway of blood cell differentiation in order to understand leukaemias and lymphomas, the principal malignancies of the circulatory systems. Mutation of cells in the myeloid pathway may lead to myeloid diseases such as myeloid leukaemia, whereas if the lymphoid pathway is affected,

then lymphoid disease such as lymphocytic leukaemia or the lymphomas may result. In fact, the current thinking about the lymphoid differentiation pathway is that it is perhaps no longer suitable to separate out lymphocytic leukaemias and lymphomas, because they are probably the same type of disease. The primary difference is that one manifests itself in the bone marrow and is termed leukaemia and the other manifests itself in the lymphatic system and is termed lymphoma. The World Health Organisation (WHO) recognised this reorganisation of traditional thinking in its classification of myeloid and lymphoid neoplasms.

TABLE 2.1	**Blood Cells and Their Function**		
Differentiation Pathway	**Cell Type**		**Role Function**
Lymphoid cells	Lymphocytes	Agranulocytes	T, B NK cells – major role in immune response; produce antibodies
Myeloid cells	Monocytes		Macrophages, ingest micro-organisms and detoxify cells; can become dendritic cell
	Eosinophils	Granulocytes (Granules in cytoplasm)	Releases toxins that kill bacteria, cause tissue damage and initiates repair
	Basophils		Releases histamine. Defence against parasites
	Mast cell		Dilates blood vessels and induces inflammation. Releases histamine and heparin. Involved in wound healing and pathogen defence by recruiting phagocytes.
	Neutrophils		Migrate into tissue, ingest and digest bacteria
	Erythrocytes (red blood cell)		Carry oxygen around the body in the form of oxy-haemoglobin, and return carbon dioxide to lungs to be excreted
	Thrombocytes (platelets)		One of several clotting factors; assist in stopping bleeding

The Lymphatic System

The lymphatic system is a specialised section of the circulatory system. Each organ in the body has an associated lymphatic drainage, the function of which is to return proteins, fats and other substances from the tissues where they have been used back to the general circulation. The lymphatic system itself is made up mainly of lymphatic vessels that are similar in structure to veins, although their walls are thinner. These vessels originate as blind-ended vessels in tissue spaces and join together to form ever larger lymphatic vessels. All the lymph eventually drains into two major lymphatic vessels: the right lymphatic duct, which receives lymph from the upper right quadrant of the body, and the thoracic duct, which receives the rest of the body's lymphatic fluid. Lymph is finally returned to the blood via the right and left subclavian veins.

As lymph is transported throughout the body it travels through oval-shaped lymph nodes. Most lymph nodes are found in groups around the body (Fig. 2.3A). Lymph nodes are enclosed by a fibrous capsule. They receive lymph from a number of afferent vessels and allow lymph to leave the node via one or two efferent vessels (see Fig. 2.3B). Valves within the lymphatic vessels allow the lymph to flow in one direction only. Trabeculae within the node form a fine meshwork of fibres which trap any harmful microorganisms contained within the lymph fluid. Throughout the cortex of the node are germinal centres that produce lymphocytes, which then act as a defence against any unwanted organisms caught within the framework.

In addition to the lymphatic vessels and lymph nodes, the body contains diffuse areas of lymphatic tissue called aggregated lymphatic nodules. These are primarily found where the body's internal environment is in contact with the external environment (e.g. in the digestive tract, where the tonsils and the aggregated lymphatic nodules in the stomach and intestines act as defences against ingested pathogens). Lymphatic tissue can also be found in the lungs and the brain.

How organs drain via the lymphatic system is important in understanding the spread of cancer in

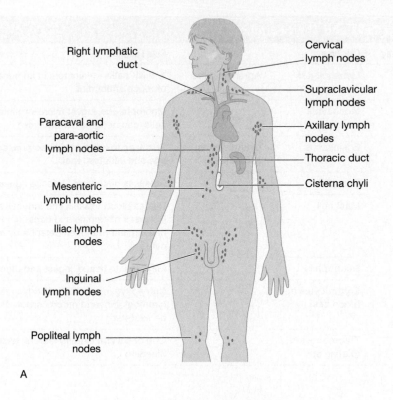

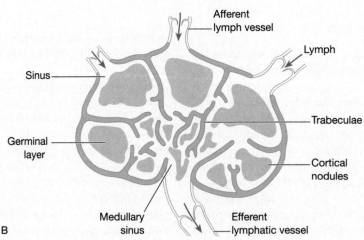

Fig. 2.3 (A) Distribution of lymph nodes; (B) a lymph node.

general. The lymphatic spread of cancer can be traced by following the lymphatic flow because lymph flows in only one direction. This is particularly important in the understanding of lymphomas, the general term to describe cancerous changes in lymphatic tissue.

Leukaemia

Leukaemia is a group of diseases characterised by the over-production of blood cells, mainly white blood cells. As mentioned earlier, we distinguish myeloid neoplasms and lymphoid neoplasms. These can be further divided into two types: acute disease leukaemia and chronic leukaemia. Acute leukaemia is typified by the presence of primitive blast cells in the bone marrow and peripheral blood. These cells are immature and at the beginning of the differentiation pathway shown in Fig. 2.2. Chronic leukaemia is associated with more mature cells that are further along the differentiation pathway but are still abnormal. The overproduction of these abnormal blood cells, again usually white cells, crowds out other blood cells, usually red blood cells and platelets. This leads to the common presenting symptoms such as anaemia and a tendency to bleed or bruise easily. In leukaemia, because only one type of white blood cell is being overproduced, other white blood cells, such as neutrophils, may be under-produced. Because of this and also because the abnormal white blood cells do not function properly, the patient is susceptible to infection, which is one of the main causes of death, along with total bone marrow failure.

A variety of aetiologic factors have been associated with leukaemia. It can be caused by ionising radiation and also by cytotoxic chemotherapy (alkylating agents and topoisomerase II inhibitors), although there is scant evidence to suggest that the two together have a synergistic effect. Some industrial chemicals such as benzene are implicated in acute myeloblastic leukaemia. A genetic aetiologic factor in leukaemia has also been suggested. People with Down syndrome have a higher risk of leukaemia, approximately 90% of chronic myeloid leukaemia cases are associated with the Philadelphia chromosome (Ph) (resulting from a translocation between chromosomes 9 and 22) and the *PML/RARA* fusion gene is responsible for acute promyelocytic leukaemia (APL), an aggressive form of acute myeloid leukaemia (AML). Such knowledge of these 'fusion' genes has led to a more directed (targeted) approach to treatments with a good deal of success. Furthermore, the Epstein–Barr virus (EBV) has been associated with haematopoietic disease of the lymphoid series.

Acute and chronic haematopoietic disease, having been further subdivided by their differentiation pathways (lymphoid or myeloid), can be grouped together to form four major disease categories:

- acute lymphoblastic leukaemia (ALL)
- acute myeloblastic leukaemia

- chronic lymphocytic leukaemia (CLL)
- chronic myelogenous (or myeloid, or granulocytic) leukaemia (CML).

Myeloid leukaemias may sometimes be referred to as granulocytic or myelocytic. Lymphoid leukaemias may be further subdivided into T and B cell types. Note that the terminology used here describes where the malignant cell is on the differentiation pathway. For example, myeloblastic indicates that the malignant cell is an immature myelocyte at the beginning of the differentiation pathway. Lymphocytic indicates that the malignant cell is a mature lymphocyte towards the end of the differentiation pathway.

ACUTE MYELOID LEUKAEMIA

AML is a rare disease which mainly affects adults older than 40 years. Rates are slightly higher in males, and although direct aetiology is not known, prior exposure to radiation has been associated with onset of the disease. Smokers are at higher risk, mainly due to the inhalation of benzene, a by-product of tobacco leaf combustion. Benzene is also found in cleaning products, solvents and rubber production, and overexposure increases the risk of AML in people who work in these industries. Furthermore, people who have been treated for an initial cancer with alkylating agent chemotherapy or topoisomerase II inhibitors have an increased risk of AML. AML can be preceded by myelodysplastic syndrome (MDS), a condition which manifests itself in low levels of all blood cells, which can evolve over time into AML. Certain other blood conditions, myeloproliferative diseases such as polycythaemia rubra vera, essential thrombocythemia and idiopathic myelofibrosis also increase the risk of AML, and more so if they have been treated with chemotherapy.

Presenting symptoms for AML are generally associated with a decrease in functioning blood cells leading to tiredness, generalised infections and bleeding/bruising. Patients may also experience a build-up of leukaemic cells in joints, leading to joint pain and stiffness. Furthermore, although not common, infiltration of the central nervous system (CNS), where leukaemic cells can find sanctuary, may occur.

AML is diagnosed by bone marrow aspirate, which identifies more than 20% blast cells, although if a chromosomal abnormality is present, diagnosis may be made with less than 20%. Investigating chromosomal abnormalities and gene mutations, as well as certain protein expression, is an integral part of the classification of AML and indeed has led to the development of more targeted therapies with positive clinical results.

In general, AML is classified using the WHO system, although the older, more traditional French–American–British (FAB) system may also be used. The WHO pays more attention to the genetic variation of AML and furthermore describes three categories:

1. AML with genetic abnormalities (e.g. APL (*PML/RARA* fusion gene) and t(8:21))
2. AML with myelodysplasia-related changes
3. tAML related to previous treatment with chemotherapy or radiation.

Gene mutations can have a bearing on prognosis and treatment; for example, mutation in the *FLT3* gene is associated with poorer prognosis, and *FLT3*-directed therapies such as midostaurin (Rydapt) have recently been developed.

TREATMENT

Treatment for AML generally consists of two (sometimes three) stages. The first, induction, aims to get the patient into remission – that is, destroy all (or at least most) of the leukaemia cells. Intensive chemotherapy with drugs such as cytarabine and daunorubicin in combination are used to achieve this. Further chemotherapy can be over given several cycles to consolidate the remission and 'mop up' any residual disease. Intrathecal chemotherapy may be used if involvement of the CNS is demonstrated or likely.

The best chance of cure for patients is a stem cell transplant, but this would be offered only to those who are fit enough to withstand this very intensive treatment.

For patients whose leukaemia demonstrates *FLT3* gene mutation, midostaurin may be offered alongside the induction chemotherapy. Most myeloid blast cells express the CD33 protein on the cell surface. CD33 expression diminishes with cell maturation, making CD33 a good target for AML. Those patients whose disease expresses the CD33 protein might be given gemtuzumab ozogamicin (Mylotarg). Gemtuzumab ozogamicin is an antibody–drug conjugate (ADC) which uses the targeting nature of the monoclonal antibody to seek out CD33 on the leukaemic cells. Once binding has occurred, the ADC is brought into the cell, where it releases a chemotherapy payload and initiates cell death.

One notable subtype of AML is APL (M3 in the FAB classification) and is diagnosed through demonstration of the *PML/RARA* fusion gene, generally caused by a translocation between chromosome 15 and 17, t(15:17). The resultant *PML/RARA* fusion gene halts differentiation of these myeloid cells in the 'blast' phase of development. APL results from over-production of these cells. All-trans retinoic acid (ATRA), vitamin A, is used to 'force' these cells to mature and fully differentiate and eventually die. ATRA may be given alongside arsenic trioxide, and together they have improved the outcome significantly for patients with APL. Just a note of caution: Forcing these cells in maturation may produce a side effect known as 'differentiation syndrome' caused by cytokine release from abundant maturing myelocytes. Such a syndrome presents symptoms such as dyspnoea, fever, weight gain, peripheral oedema and, on rare occasions, blood clotting and/or severe bleeding. Differentiation syndrome is usually treated with steroids.

CHRONIC MYELOID LEUKAEMIA

A disease affecting people around 60 years of age, CML (or myeloid, or granulocytic leukaemia) is of particular interest to oncologists because it is associated with a specific genetic abnormality. In approximately 95% of cases, the leukaemic cells display a chromosomal abnormality associated with a translocation of cytogenetic material between the long arms of chromosomes 9 and 22, t(9:22). The resultant chromosome is called the Ph chromosome, or *BCR/ABL1* gene, and is the driving force behind CML. The onset of the disease is slow, as the disease progresses through a chronic phase, and many people may present incidentally. Symptoms associated with decreased levels of blood cells ensue; thrombocytopaenia (bruising, bleeding), anaemia (tiredness, lethargy) and neutropenia (infections) are common presenting symptoms, and the patient may experience severe splenomegaly and a significantly elevated white cell count. The chronic phase of the disease will eventually transform into an accelerated and subsequently blastic phase, which is typified by increased numbers of immature blast cells in the bone marrow. Transformation into the accelerated and blastic phases tends to be associated with poorer prognosis.

TABLE 2.2 Acute Versus Chronic Myeloid Leukaemia	
Acute Myeloid Leukaemia	**Chronic Myeloid Leukaemia**
Mainly adult (40–60 years) – 80%	Philadelphia chromosome (Ph+) (95%)
>20% blast cells (all sorts)	30–80 years (55 years)
t(8:21) and t(15:17) – Auer rods	Mature cells
Crowding out symptoms	Lots of white blood cells – mainly granulocytes
tAML	Enlarged organs and crowding out
Anthracycline (daunorubicin and cytarabine)	Pruritus (↑ basophils)
ATRA for t(15:17) (M3)	Asymptomatic (20%–40%)
Intrathecal chemotherapy for children	Chronic → accelerated → blastic
Possible stem cell transplant	Palliation, watch and wait
	Imatinib (first line), nilotinib (second)

ATRA, All-trans retinoic acid.

TREATMENT

The Ph chromosome, or *BCR/ABL1* gene, switches on messages within the white blood cells which promote growth and proliferation of these mature-looking cells. *BCR/ABL1* gene is a tyrosine kinase; kinases are a 'doing' protein and in this case promote cell growth as suggested. Using this knowledge, scientists have developed tyrosine kinase inhibitors (TKIs) to combat the working of this gene. Imatinib (Glivec, Gleevec) is a first-generation inhibitor of the *BCR/ABL1* gene and stops the growth message. Imatinib is now seen as the first-line treatment for people in the chronic phase of CML, and many patients will see long-term responses lasting many years. The drug can also be used within the accelerated and blastic phases but to less good effect. Most patients will experience some side effects – diarrhoea, nausea, muscle pain, fatigue and, in rare cases, oedema. Sometimes these side effects are deemed intolerable by the patient or the disease becomes resistant to imatinib. In such cases, other TKIs such as dasatinib are used as a first-line treatment for those who cannot tolerate imatinib or as a second-line treatment when imatinib stops working. Other TKIs might include nilotinib, bosutinib or ponatinib. Table 2.2 outlines the differences between ALL and CLL.

LYMPHOCYTIC LEUKAEMIA

The term lymphocytic leukaemia describes neoplasms that manifest in the bone marrow, and this differentiates this type of disease from lymphomas, which present as a disease of the lymphatic system. Lymphocytic leukaemia can be subcategorised as acute or chronic and may be of B cell or T cell origin.

ACUTE LYMPHOBLASTIC LEUKAEMIA

ALL is a disease of malignant lymphoblasts and immature lymphocytes; it affects mainly children and is one of the most common forms of cancer in childhood. It normally presents between 2 and 8 years of age, with peak incidence at 4 years. There is a slightly higher incidence among boys. Most symptoms are due to infiltration of the bone marrow, causing anaemia, thrombocytopenia, bone pain and infection. Enlargement of lymph nodes, splenomegaly and hepatomegaly may also be present. Rarely, the patient may present with involvement of the CNS meninges, which may cause headaches and vomiting.

Diagnostic investigation may include bone marrow aspiration and full (complete) blood count. The aim is to detect increased levels of lymphoblasts. Normally, an elevated white blood count is seen, but this may not always be the case. ALL is essentially classified according to the cell type involved, either B or T lymphocytes, and whether certain genetic abnormalities exist. Certain of these abnormalities might indicate specific treatments (e.g. imatinib might be added to treatment for Ph-positive ALL) or indeed give an indication of prognosis (e.g. patients with disease that demonstrates a translocation between chromosome 4 and 11, t(4:11) tend to have a worse prognosis and therefore might warrant more intensive treatment if possible). In general, the earlier in the B cell lineage and the younger the patient, the better the prognosis. Patients presenting with T cell leukaemia tend to be male and older than other ALL patients, and they often present with an enlarged thymus gland (diagnosed on x-ray) which may cause breathing problems and in rare cases obstruction of the superior vena cava.

Treatment of childhood ALL consists of three distinct phases that may take as long as 2 to 3 years to complete.

Induction – This first phase involves intensive chemotherapy with the aim of inducing remission of the disease, usually a combination of vincristine, prednisone and L-asparaginase. The aim is to get the peripheral blood cell counts to return to near normal. Intrathecal methotrexate will also be used, either because there is evidence of CNS involvement or as prophylaxis to reduce the chance of CNS involvement. Ph-positive patients may also receive imatinib (Glivec). Induction will be successful in 95% of patients.

Consolidation – This next phase is a relatively short phase designed to mop up any unidentified leukaemic cells that might still be present. Typical drug combinations include methotrexate, 6-mercaptopurine (6-MP), vincristine, L-asparaginase and/or prednisone, and CNS treatment may continue, as well as imatinib for those with Ph-positive disease.

Maintenance usually consists of oral 6-MP and oral methotrexate for up to 3 years after remission. In boys, there is a chance of relapse in the testes, another leukaemic sanctuary site. This can be confirmed at biopsy, and the affected testis removed. Testicular radiation may also be administered.

ACUTE LYMPHOBLASTIC LEUKAEMIA IN ADULTS

The clinical presentation of adult patients is similar to that described earlier, but a higher proportion will present with a mediastinal mass. Approximately 30% of cases are Ph positive, and this is usually associated with poorer prognosis. Morphologically, the disease is classified similar to childhood ALL. The treatment of adult ALL is like the treatment of childhood ALL, although the chemotherapy regimens at remission and consolidation stages may be more intense. Intrathecal methotrexate is used to treat the cerebrospinal axis.

Patients who relapse and are fit enough may be offered a stem cell transplant. Other more novel treatments also exist in this relapsed setting. Blinatumomab is a bispecific monoclonal antibody designed to target the CD19 protein, which can be found on the surface of B cells and also attaches to the CD3 protein found on T cells. Such an approach is designed to bring immune cells and cancer cells close together and initiate tumour cell destruction. Another approach which has been trialled for patients where other therapies have failed uses chimeric antigen receptor T cells, or CAR(T), a novel approach which uses genetically modified T cells which recognise tumour cell proteins. The T cells are multiplied in the laboratory then given back to the patient. Such an approach unleashes an immune attack on the targeted cells. However, such an approach is suitable only for those fit enough to withstand the side effects associated. Cytokine release syndrome is a common occurrence which can manifest in a wide range of symptoms such as fever, chills, nausea, confusion, headaches and loss of balance. Some of these effects can be life-changing and/or life-threatening.

In general, approximately 85% of adults with ALL will achieve remission, with this percentage being higher in children. Approximately 40% to 50% of adults will survive more than 5 years, with the percentage being approximately 90% for children.

CHRONIC LYMPHOCYTIC LEUKAEMIA

CLL generally affects people older than 50 years; it is the most common type of adult leukaemia and is slightly more common in males. The onset of the disease is insidious; approximately 25% of patients are diagnosed incidentally on routine blood tests or medical examination. Common symptoms include anaemia and enlargement of lymph nodes. The spleen may also be enlarged, although not to the same extent as in CML. Very elevated white cell counts (leucocytosis) are common. Often this disease is grouped together with low-grade non-Hodgkin small lymphocytic lymphoma because it is now recognised that the B lymphocyte is the malignant cell and only the background tissue (bone marrow in leukaemia versus lymph nodes in lymphoma) is different and in later stages may involve generalised lymphadenopathy.

TREATMENT

Prior to any treatment, decisions are usually made regarding the intended outcome. There is no known treatment that can cure this disease; however, patients

TABLE 2.3	Staging Systems for Chronic Lymphocytic Leukaemia
(a) Binet staging	
A	No anaemia or thrombocytopenia and fewer than three areas of lymphoid involvement
B	No anaemia or thrombocytopenia with three or more areas of lymphoid involvement
C	Anaemia and/or thrombocytopenia regardless of the number of areas of lymphoid enlargement
(b) Rai staging system	
0	Lymphocytosis (>15,000/mm^3) **without** lymphadenopathy, hepatosplenomegaly, anaemia or thrombocytopenia
I	Lymphocytosis **with** lymphadenopathy **but without** hepatosplenomegaly, anaemia or thrombocytopenia
II	Lymphocytosis with **either** hepatomegaly or splenomegaly **with or without** lymphadenopathy
III	Lymphocytosis **and** anaemia (haemoglobin <11 g/dL) **with or without** lymphadenopathy, hepatomegaly or splenomegaly
IV	Lymphocytosis **and** thrombocytopenia (<100,000/mm^3) **with or without** lymphadenopathy, hepatomegaly, splenomegaly or anaemia

Binet stage A and Rai stage 0/I would be considered indolent, slow-growing disease. As such, treatment may be delayed until such time as symptoms become troublesome. Treatment intervention may earlier with more aggressive forms such as Binet stage C or Rai stage III/IV.

can often live for many years with no therapy. Whether or not to administer treatment will depend on certain factors.

Age – Most patients will be older than 50 years. The age, along with comorbidity, might preclude certain types of aggressive treatment, and given the slow nature of the disease in most cases, risk might outweigh any benefit.

Staging – Two staging systems exist (Table 2.3). The Rai staging system is mainly used in the United States, whereas the Binet staging system is more often used in Europe.

Genetic abnormalities – Research has begun to demonstrate certain genetic abnormalities that may be/are useful as prognostic indicators and may lead to better stratification of treatments. For example, some malignant cells might demonstrate mutation in the *IgVH* gene. Point of note here. Normal B cells undergo maturation to become a mature B cell. The purpose of a B cell (mainly) is to produce antibodies. Antibodies, or immunoglobulins (Igs), help to fight infection, and to produce these antibodies the B cell must undergo certain changes (mutations) as it matures. These changes, mutations, are a normal process that the B cell undergoes to become a fully differentiated B cell which can do its job—produce antibodies. The *IgVH* gene is an important part of this process, and when it is mutated, it means that the B cell is mature and able to produce antibodies. In this sense the mutated *IgVH* is a positive thing and demonstrates the CLL cells are more mature and tend to be slow growing. Such an indication might help in decisions about treatment, and mutated *IgVH* is associated with better prognosis than if the *IgVH* gene is unmutated.

Two other genetic 'fingerprints' may help with decisions about prognosis and treatment. Over-expression of the ZAP-70 and/or CD38 proteins may have an impact on survival. Recent studies have suggested that low levels of these proteins on the cell surface (ZAP-70 <20%; CD38 <30%) tend to be associated with better long-term survival.

Furthermore, expression of the CD20 protein is useful for adding rituximab to any chemotherapy; mutated BTK (Bruton tyrosine kinase), a protein which promotes growth and survival, might indicate the use of ibrutinib, a BTK blocker, and, similarly, mutated P13K might indicate treatment with idelalisib.

TABLE 2.4 Differences Between Acute and Chronic Lymphoblastic Leukaemia	
Acute Lymphoblastic Leukaemia (ALL)	**Chronic Lymphocytic Leukaemia (CLL)**
2–8 years (mainly) (– adult Ph+)	30% of leukaemias, T or B
Tiredness, lymphadenopathy, crowding out	Cross over with NHL
↑↑ Blast cells, enlarged organs, bone pain	M:F 2:1: >50 years
B (CD10,19) or T (CD2,5,7)	Full Blood Count – lymphocytosis with possible smudge cells
Remission (vincristine, asparaginase, prednisolone)	Low ZAP-70 & CD38 better prognosis
Consolidation and maintenance	Immunoincompetent cells → infections, bleeding, night sweats
Intrathecal methotrexate	Tiredness, ↑ spleen
+++ Survival	25% incidental findings
	Watch and wait
	FCR (fludarabine, cyclophosphamide, rituximab)
	CHOP
	BTK, P13K, BCL2 mutations possible

BTK, Bruton tyrosine kinase; *CHOP*, cyclophosphamide, doxorubicin, vincristine, prednisolone; *NHL*, non-Hodgkin lymphoma.

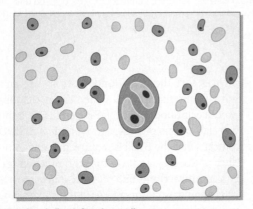

Fig. 2.4 Classic Reed–Sternberg cell.

Many patients will be asymptomatic at presentation and, as such, will fall into the 'wait and wait' category of management. Once symptoms become troublesome, active treatment might ensue, considering factors as discussed previously. Chemotherapy, if used, would generally include fludarabine with rituximab and maybe cyclophosphamide. Stem cell transplant may be an option for those fit enough.

A point of note: In approximately 5% to 10% of cases, CLL may undergo a transformation into a lymphoma. This is referred to as a Richter transformation, and the disease begins to behave more like and be treated like diffuse large B cell lymphoma (DLBCL; more said about this later).

Table 2.4 outlines the differences between ALL and CLL.

Overall, the prognosis is better for younger people who can withstand the intensive treatments required. However, improvement in the detection of genetic subtypes in leukaemia has led to a more targeted approach to treatment. As stated earlier, imatinib (Glivec) has changed the landscape for those with CML, and ATRA is proven to be a particularly good treatment for many with APL. Applying potentially different treatments to different subtypes of leukaemia may help to improve treatment for those with that genetic subtype, which in the long term will improve survival in adult leukaemia across the board.

LYMPHOMAS

ONCOLOGY

Lymphomas can occur anywhere in the body where there is lymphatic tissue. The two main types of lymphoma are Hodgkin lymphoma (HL) and non-Hodgkin lymphoma (NHL). HL mainly affects the lymph nodes, and NHL can affect the diffuse lymphatic tissues throughout the body, although lymph node involvement may occur also.

HODGKIN LYMPHOMA

With conventional therapies, HL is highly curable. A better understanding of how the lymphatic system functions and better staging techniques, along with a greater understanding of how radiotherapy and chemotherapy work, have resulted in considerable success in the management of patients with this type of lymphoma.

The incidence of HL is bimodal. It is rare to develop the disease younger than 5 years of age. There is a major peak around 15 to 25 years and a further peak in middle age. HL is slightly more common in males. Although a direct aetiologic link is unknown, the majority of cases are associated with EBV. The disease is characterised by the presence of atypical, multinucleated Reed–Sternberg (RS) cells (Fig. 2.4), which replace normal lymphocytes in the lymphatic tissue. RS cells originate from germinal centre B cells and are malignant portion of HL. Classic RS cells typically have the 'owl-eye' appearance seen in Fig. 2.4 and are more often found in the mixed cell type of HL; other types such as Lacunar-type RS cells, so called because the single nucleus is surrounded by clear cytoplasm, is more often found in the nodular sclerosing variety. In addition, pleomorphic RS cells, which demonstrate atypical nuclei of different sizes and shapes, are present in lymphocyte-depleted HL. Pathologic testing for these varieties will help with the subclassification of this disease. Furthermore, through immunohistocytochemistry testing, the RS cell will be CD15+ and CD30+.

On presentation, patients generally have enlarged lymph nodes in the cervical region, axilla or supraclavicular regions. This adenopathy differs from the enlargement of normal nodes as a result of infection, in that the nodes appear more rubbery and firm in HL. The classification of HL can be seen in Table 2.5. Please note two distinct varieties: classical HL and nodular lymphocyte predominance. The notable difference is that the RS cells in the latter tend to be CD20+ and will be CD15− and CD30−, thereby classifying it as a separate entity. CD20 is a target for the drug rituximab. Successful multiagent chemotherapy regimens mean that histologic subtype tends not to influence outcome for patients with HL.

STAGING

Typically, the spread of HL follows the route of the lymphatics from where the disease originated. It is rare for HL to skip lymph node stations and is said to be 'contiguous'. Therefore, knowledge of the lymphatic drainage for areas of the body is crucial in understanding the likely spread of HL. The favoured staging system is the Ann Arbor staging system (Table 2.6). Accurate staging of the disease influences the treatment of patients with HL. The advent of positron emission tomography (PET) scans has led to even more accurate localisation of disease, with better staging prospects.

TABLE 2.5   Histological Variations of Hodgkin Lymphoma

Name		Description
Nodular sclerosing	Classical Hodgkin Lymphoma	Is the most common subtype, lacuna-type Reed–Sternberg (RS) cells in a background of inflammatory cells with varying degrees of collagen fibrosis/*sclerosis*.
Mixed cellularity		Common subtype, numerous classic RS cells mixed with numerous inflammatory without sclerosis. Most often associated with Epstein–Barr virus infection.
Lymphocyte rich		Rare subtype, show many features which may cause diagnostic confusion with nodular lymphocyte-predominant B-NHL. Most favourable prognosis.
Lymphocyte depleted		Rare subtype, large numbers of often pleomorphic RS cells with only few reactive lymphocytes. Poor prognosis.
Nodular lymphocyte-predominant		Presence of popcorn cells or 'polypoid' RS cells. Large multilobed nucleus which resemble popcorn. Good prognosis, slow-growing, but may recur.

TABLE 2.6   Ann Arbor Staging for Hodgkin Lymphoma

Stage	Description
I	Involvement of a single lymph region (I) or a single extralymphatic organ (IE)
II	Involvement of two or more lymph node regions on the same side of the diaphragm (II) or localised involvement of an extralymphatic organ or site and of one or more lymph node regions on the same side of the diaphragm (IIE)
III	Involvement of lymph node regions on both sides of the diaphragm (III) which may also be accompanied by localised involvement of an extralymphatic organ or site (IIIE) or by involvement of the spleen (IIIS) or both (IIIES)
IV	Diffuse or disseminated involvement of one or more extralymphatic organs or tissues with or without associated lymph node enlargement

Furthermore, PET scans can be used to monitor the effects of treatment (chemotherapy), with the prospect of limiting the amount of chemotherapy required.

Stages I, II, III and IV HL are subclassified into A and B categories and subcategories E or S. The E subscript represents extranodal involvement, and the S subscript represents involvement of the spleen. In terms of symptoms, A is used for those patients who are asymptomatic, and B is used for those patients with any of the following specific symptoms:

- unexplained weight loss (more than 10% of body weight)
- unexplained fever for more than 3 days
- drenching night sweats.

The presence of B symptoms may indicate that the patient has systemic disease even though it may not be evident from clinical staging. Patients with B symptoms are treated with systemic chemotherapy rather than localised radiotherapy.

Stage IV may be further annotated with the following to define the extralymphatic organ involved: L, lung; M, bone marrow; O, osseous; P, pleura; H, hepatic; D, derma; S, spleen.

TREATMENT

Modern treatment for classical HL has led to long-term cure in the majority of patients. Chemotherapy with the drug combination ABVD (adriamycin (doxorubicin), bleomycin, vinblastine, dacarbazine (DTIC)) is the treatment of choice with or without localised radiotherapy to the affected lymph node groups.

Point of note. Adriamycin (doxorubicin) is an anthracycline chemotherapy drug and is known to be cardiotoxic, whilst bleomycin is pneumotoxic and vincristine is neurotoxic. Hence, it is advantageous to limit the amount given. PET scans are often retaken after three or four cycles of ABVD. If the disease is in remission, then chemotherapy might be halted, thus limiting the possibilities of further long-term side effects. Older persons with HL with comorbidity such as heart disease may be offered ChlVPP (chlorambucil, vincristine, procarbazine, prednisolone) as an alternative regimen.

For those whose disease relapses, brentuximab vedotin (Adcetris) is an option. This ADC uses the targeting nature of the monoclonal antibody to attached to CD30, which is present on RS cells. Once attached, it is taken into the cell, where it deposits an antimitotic agent (MMAE – monomethyl auristatin (Vedotin)), which kills the cell. Stem cell transplants remain an option for those fit enough for the procedure.

Nodular lymphocyte-predominant HL is a particular subtype which is very slow-growing and rarely fatal, although it can recur. This disease can still be classed as HL because of the presence of RS cells. However, these RS cells will be CD15– and CD30– (note: classical HL is positive for these), and it will be CD20+. Consequently, if treatment is offered (many patients will just be monitored), CHOP-R (cyclophosphamide, doxorubicin, vincristine, prednisolone, rituximab) likely will be used. Note that rituximab is a monoclonal antibody which targets CD20 and signals the cell for immune destruction.

NON-HODGKIN LYMPHOMA

NHL is a general term used to describe a heterogeneous group of malignant disorders that mainly occur in older age groups. Presenting symptoms may be similar to those of HL, although it is more likely that disease involves extranodal or extralymphatic sites. The patient often presents with already disseminated disease and B symptoms. Although the aetiology of NHL is unknown, the risk of a person developing NHL is increased in immunodeficiency disorders. RS cells are not present in NHL. Certain NHLs, such

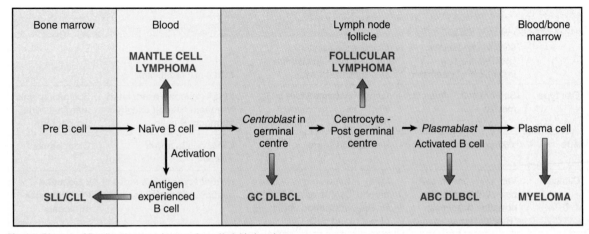

Fig. 2.5 Diagram of B cell pathway and types of non-Hodgkin lymphoma.

as Burkitt lymphoma, are associated with EBV, especially in African children, in whom the disease is more common. NHL is an overproliferation of B cells or T cells – lymphocytes that have different differentiation pathways – thus, there are many forms and names of lymphoma.

Before T and B lymphocytes can fully differentiate (i.e. become a mature functioning T or B cell), they must undergo a process of recognition. The role of both these cells, albeit through different mechanisms, is to recognise and destroy invaders to the body, (antigens).

T cells are formed in the bone marrow and migrate to the thymus in foetal life. They differentiate into a range of T cells with differing functions, including helper T cells, suppressor T cells, memory T cells and killer T cells. These then migrate to lymph nodes and lodge in the paracortical region of the lymph node. B cells are formed in the bone marrow and from there migrate to the lymph nodes where they lodge in the follicle of the lymph node, which contains a germinal centre and an outer margin. Eventually, B cells will become either a memory B cell or a plasma cell, which will generate antibodies against the invading antigen. See Fig. 2.5, which outlines the maturation and activation pathway of B cells and how this relates to the types of NHL.

To mature, the B cell needs to undergo many somatic (self-induced) genetic changes; this is referred to as 'somatic hypermutation', and the net result is

a series of changes within the cell's DNA which will allow it to make the antibodies required. There are many more B cell lymphomas than there are T cell, lymphomas, likely because the B cell needs to undergo all these genetic changes to mature and is therefore more susceptible to things going wrong.

As well as separating NHL into T or B cell lymphoma, it is also useful to separate them according to their grade, either low grade or high grade.

LOW-GRADE NON-HODGKIN LYMPHOMA

Such lymphomas tend to be very slow-growing, matur(ish) B cells. The most common type is follicular lymphoma, which derives from the post–germinal centre B cell (centrocyte) and is associated with a translocation between chromosome 14 and chromosome 18, t(14:18). Such a translocation upregulates the *BCL2* gene, which in turn blocks apoptosis (programmed cell death), which allows these defective cells to continue growth and proliferation. Because these cells are more mature, they will tend to arrange themselves like normal B cells and form the follicle- type structures found in the normal architecture of a lymph node; hence the term follicular lymphoma.

The nature of these types of lymphoma, their well-differentiated appearance and indolent presentation mean that many patients will present with late-stage disease. In addition, the slow nature of the disease means that, although responsive to chemotherapy, it

TABLE 2.7   Low-Grade Non-Hodgkin Lymphoma

	Chronic Lymphocytic Leukaemia/Small Lymphocytic Lymphoma	Lymphoplasmacyctic Lymphoma (Waldenström Macroglobulinaemia)	Extranodal Lymphoma	
Cell type	Small B cell, diffuse but mature	Lymphoplasmacytoid cells (B cell in the process of maturing)	MALT (mucosa-associated lymphoid tissue); usually stomach; B cells	Splenic (splenic marginal zone lymphoma)
Age	>60 years	V rare; >60 years	Older adults (more women)	Older adults
Clinical	Very slow onset; sple-nomegaly; lymphade-nopathy; tiredness; *Richter transformation	Ig(M) → hyperviscosity (nose bleeds, confusion, vision) Rouleux formation (stacking) of red blood cells	*Helicobacter pylori;* indi-gestion, abdominal pain	? Hepatitis C infection; sple-nomegaly
Treatment	Watch & wait; FCR (fludarabine, cyclo-phosphamide, ritux-imab); **alemtuzumab (Campath)	Plasmapheresis, chlorambucil	Antibiotics; may be fol-lowed by RT or CT	Watch & wait; splenectomy

CT, Chemotherapy; *RT*, radiotherapy.
* Richter transformation: cells become larger and immature. They divide more often and the lymphoma is said to have transformed to high grade.
** Alemtuzumab targets CD52. A surface protein on mature B cells. Targets them for destruction, and new cells produced.
NOTE: All patients with relapsed low grade NHL may be offered Stem cell transplants if fit enough

is often difficult to irradicate the disease entirely and many patients' disease will have a typically relapsing and remitting course, meaning that it will come back at some point. Many of these cells will exhibit the CD20 marker on their cell surface. CD20 is the tar-get for the drug rituximab, which will be given along with the chemotherapy. Table 2.7 outlines some of the other less common types of low-grade NHL.

HIGH-GRADE NON-HODGKIN LYMPHOMA

High-grade NHLs tend to be faster growing, be aggres-sive and involve other parts of the body, such as the bone marrow, quicker. The cells will be poorly differ-entiated and will not behave like normal, and the cells will be spread out (i.e. diffuse rather than making any of the normal structures, as mentioned earlier). The fast-growing nature means that they respond well, in most cases, to treatments such as chemotherapy. The most common type of high-grade NHL is DLBCL, of which there are two main types: germinal centre–like DLBCL and activated B cell–like DLBCL (a third type, thymic B cell lymphoma, also exists). These subtypes

are important because they may respond differently to the chemotherapy currently on offer for these patients. Table 2.8 shows some of the other less common high-grade lymphomas.

STAGING

The staging system for NHL is similar to that for HL, the Ann Arbor. Noncontiguous lymph node involve-ment, which is uncommon in HL, is more common among patients with NHL. Extralymphatic involve-ment of the gastrointestinal tract, brain, uterus and breast is also more common. A single extranodal or extralymphatic site is occasionally the only site of involvement in patients with diffuse lymphoma. Bone marrow and hepatic involvement are especially com-mon in patients with low-grade lymphomas, and cyto-logical examination of cerebrospinal fluid (CSF) may be positive in patients with aggressive NHL.

TREATMENT

The treatment of NHL depends in large part on the histological type, location and stage of the disease, as

TABLE 2.8 High-Grade Non-Hodgkin Lymphoma

	Burkitt Lymphoma	Lymphoblastic Lymphoma	Adult T Cell Leukaemia/ Lymphoma
Cell type	B cell • Endemic variant (also called "African variant") – Epstein–Barr virus (EBV) • Sporadic – not EBV • Immunodeficiency-associated (HIV/AIDS, post transplants)	T (mainly) or B cells Very similar too acute lymphoblastic leukaemia (ALL) and can transform	T cells
Aetiology/age	Young (one-third of lymphomas in children)	Mainly children	50–60 years Asian, African, Caribbean origin Associated with HTLV-1
Clinical	• t(8:14) → over-active cMyc in 95% of cases • Tend to be aggressive and widespread, including extranodal sites • Commonly affects central nervous system (CNS)	Can affect CNS and Skin and typically thymus (mediastinum)	Enlarged nodes Bone marrow involvement Hypercalcaemia Hepatosplenomegaly Skin involvement
Treatment	CODOX-M/IVAC	Chemotherapy Remission Consolidation Maintenance CNS prophylaxis	Alpha-interferon CHOP

CHOP, Cyclophosphamide, doxorubicin, vincristine, prednisolone.

well as the general condition of the patient. However, some general principles can be applied (Table 2.9).

Histological type – follicular lymphoma is a very indolent disease: hard to cure but controllable. The presence of gene mutations *BCL2* and *BCL6* is often associated with poorer prognosis and may help in determining management. High-grade lymphoma such as DLBCL will respond much better to chemotherapy because of the rapidity of the disease. However, even here, specific genetic variations will affect outcome. For example, as outlined earlier, activated B cell–like DLBCL does not respond as well to R-CHOP as the germinal centre–like DLBCL.

General condition of the patient – treatment for NHL can be long, sometimes intensive with chemotherapy drugs that tend to have organ specific toxicity. Therefore, comorbidity needs to be taken into account. It would be difficult to give high doses of anthracycline chemotherapy if the patient has a heart condition. Performance status scales such as the Eastern Cooperative Oncology Group (ECOG)/WHO criteria or Karnofsky Criteria can help to measure a person's ability to tolerate treatment, evaluate response to treatment, assess if/how cancer is progressing and estimate prognosis.

To further stratify patients into prognostic groups, the International Prognostic Index (IPI) may be used. The IPI assigns points to five established criteria: age (<60 years 0 pts, >60 years 1 pt), lactase dehydrogenase hormone (LDH) levels (low 0 pts, high 1 pt), performance status (manage daily tasks 0 pts, needs a lot of assistance 1 pt), stage (early 0 pts, late 1 pt) and extranodal involvement (none 0 pts, involvement 1 pt). Patients with higher scores tend to have a greater chance of relapse.

POINTS TO NOTE

NHL is a heterogenous group of diseases often driven by key gene mutations and influenced by their level of differentiation. Using different criteria to assign patients to different prognostic and treatment groups allows for

TABLE 2.9		Principles of Treatment for Non-Hodgkin Lymphoma	
		Stage	
		Limited	**Advanced**
Grade	**Low**	RT to affected nodes	Watch and wait First line: R-CHOP Maintenance – Rituximab Second line – R-CHOP Or bendamustine
	High	R-CHOP ± RT to nodes Maybe intrathecal CT	R-CHOP (maybe intrathecal CT) Possible stem cell transplant if fit enough Relapse – RICE

CHOP, Cyclophosphamide, doxorubicin, vincristine, prednisolone; *CT*, chemotherapy; *RT*, radiotherapy; *R*, rituximab; *RICE*, rituximab, ifosfamide, carboplatin, etoposide.

a more personalised approach to many of the treatments on offer. Many more treatments are being developed, which leads to a rich treatment horizon, even for those patients with relapsed or refractory disease.

MYELOMA

Myeloma, or multiple myeloma, is a type of cancer originating in the bone marrow and is a result of a neoplastic change in plasma cells (see Fig. 2.2). Plasma cells are mature B lymphocytes which reside in the bone marrow and produce antibodies to help fight infection. Myeloma manifests through the over-production of one variety of plasma cell (monoclonal) and consequently leads to the over-production of the antibody with associated signs and symptoms.

Antibodies are Y-shaped (or combinations of Y-shapes) structures and are produced to combat a specific antigen; see Fig. 2.6.

Antibodies, or Igs, are large structures composed of a heavy chain, which can be G, A, M, D or E, and a light chain γ or κ, along with a variable region which is adapted to suit the respective antigen. Normally a robust structure, in myeloma, the malignant plasma cells often make fragile versions of the antibody, and the light chains in particular can break off and be detected in the blood. Such raised levels are referred to as a 'paraprotein or monoclonal spike', which is used in the diagnosis of myeloma.

Very much a disease of the older population, myeloma is rare before the age of 50 years, and although

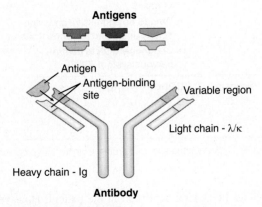

Fig. 2.6 Structure of an antibody.

the cause is largely unknown, it is twice as common in Black populations and in some cases is seen to run in families. It is thought that most myeloma will be preceded by a condition called monoclonal gammopathy of undetermined significance (MGUS), indicating an over-production of plasma cells and antibody but significantly no 'end-of-life organ' damage. Table 2.10 shows the difference in levels and symptoms associated with myeloma and other conditions.

Myeloma is currently considered an incurable disease in most cases, but with more knowledge of the myeloma microenvironment, new drugs have been developed, which leads to myeloma being a very controllable disease. Although the disease will relapse in most cases, the aim of treatment is to reduce the plasma cell burden, relieve the symptoms and

TABLE 2.10 Monoclonal Gammopathy of Undetermined Significance (MGUS) Versus Smouldering Myeloma Versus Symptomatic Myeloma and CRAB Criteria

		MGUS	Smouldering Myeloma	Symptomatic Myeloma
Plasma cells in bone marrow		<10%	≥10%	>10%
Paraprotein		<30 g/L	>30 g/L	Raised (may be in urine also)
Evidence of end of life organ damage	HyperCalcaemia	–	–	+
	Renal impairment	–	–	+
	Anaemia	–	–	+
	Bone lesions	–	–	+

complications caused by the myeloma and ultimately improve the quality and prolong the life of the patient with myeloma.

CRAB (see Table 2.10) is a useful acronym which describes the signs and symptoms associated with myeloma, and evidence of these helps in the diagnosis of symptomatic myeloma. Too many plasma cells in the bone marrow (more than 10% of the bone marrow volume) leads to crowding out of normal blood cell production and a decrease in the number of circulating red blood cells, which leads to anaemia. Furthermore, there will be a decrease in neutrophils, as well as useful Igs, which will make the patient susceptible to infections. One of the most common symptoms is lower back pain, or bone pain in general. The bone marrow stromal cells will stimulate the growth and development of the myeloma cells, which in turn secrete cytokines which will inhibit or promote the action of two further types of bone cell. Osteoblasts are bone cells responsible for the deposition of bone, and osteoclasts are responsible for the absorption of bone. These two cells work together in a constant bone remodelling process. The myeloma cells will secrete cytokines, such as interleukin-3 (IL-3) and IL-6, which will inhibit the action of osteoblasts, which, at the same time, promote the action of osteoclasts. The net result is that too much bone is eroded, which leads to two effects. Firstly, the over-erosion of the bone produces 'punched out' holes, or 'lytic' lesions within the bone, leading to bone pain and possibly pathological fractures or collapsing of the vertebra and possible spinal cord compression. Secondly, the calcium deposited

in the bone is now freed and circulates within the blood, leading to hypercalcaemia, which can lead to feelings of thirst, confusion, somnolence, bone pain, constipation, nausea and dehydration. In addition, raised levels of the paraprotein in the blood can lead to hyperviscosity syndrome in some patients. Many of the small paraproteins (light chains) may be filtered through the kidneys and cause blockages of the renal tubules, leading to damage and ultimately renal failure. These light chains may be picked up in the urine through analysis, and this is referred to as 'light chain' or 'Bence Jones' myeloma. Renal impairment will also lead to a decrease in erythropoietin, a red blood cell–stimulating hormone secreted by the kidneys. Fig. 2.7 outlines the signs and symptoms.

Typical investigations will include urine and blood tests along with a bone marrow biopsy. Electrophoresis of the urine may detect the presence of light chains to aid diagnosis. Blood tests will identify raised levels of the paraprotein but also look for evidence of end-organ damage, such as raised creatinine, which could indication renal impairment and/or raised calcium. Levels of β_2-microglobulin might be monitored, with high levels maybe indicating the need for active treatment. Bone marrow biopsy is essential for determining the levels of plasma cells present in the bone marrow. Levels higher than 10% of the volume would indicate myeloma. Skeletal x-rays will be taken if possible lytic lesions are suspected. Typical 'punched-out' holes can often be seen where osteoclastic activity has caused erosion of the bone.

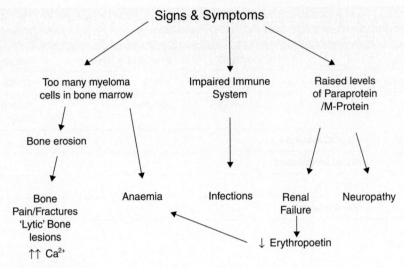

Fig. 2.7 Signs and symptoms of myeloma.

Fig. 2.8 outlines the treatment options available for most patients with myeloma and will take into consideration the age and general condition of the patient, along with any comorbidity. In general, the aim is to induce remission as quickly as possible and follow that with maintenance therapy. If the patient is fit enough, stem cells transplants are an option. A greater understanding of the myeloma microenvironment has led to a much wider range of available drugs used in different combinations, but typically a regime would include an immunomodulatory drug (IMiD) and a steroid along with either an alkylating chemotherapy agent or a proteasome inhibitor.

The myeloma cells secrete cytokines such as IL-3, IL-6 and DKK1, which promote the balance shift in bone remodelling discussed earlier, and the growth and survival of the myeloma cells. IMiDs such as thalidomide are thought to inhibit IL-6 secretion, inhibit adhesion to bone marrow stromal cells and inhibit possible angiogenesis and therefore decrease the activity and survival potential of myeloma cells.

The proteasome is a protein-recycling unit within cells which breaks down unwanted proteins produced by the cell. Antibodies, produced by plasma cells, are, in effect, long strands of protein. The myeloma cell is constantly producing antibodies, often defective and fragile, which in turn produce a lot of excess proteins that need to be recycled. Proteasome inhibitor drugs,

such as bortezomib (Velcade), inhibit the recycling unit, leading in turn to a build-up of toxic proteins within the cell, which leads to cell death.

Over-expressed target proteins on the cell surface of myeloma cells such as CD319 (target for elotuzumab) and CD38 (target for daratumumab) are useful for inducing antigen-dependent cell cytotoxicity (ADCC), where immune cells are attracted to the target and kill the myeloma cells. Recent research has also led to the use of ADCs such as belantamab mafodotin, which targets the B cell maturation antigen which is present in abundance on myeloma cells. Belantamab mafodotin uses the targeting nature of the monoclonal antibody to deliver a chemotherapy drug to the myeloma cells.

Alkylating agent chemotherapy drugs such as melphalan and cyclophosphamide have been a staple treatment for myeloma for many years, along with steroids, dexamethasone or prednisolone, and continue to play an important role; see Fig. 2.9.

In most cases, a combination of three drugs is used initially (e.g. Velcade (bortezomib), thalidomide and dexamethasone (known as VTD)), and this may be changed on relapse to melphalan, prednisolone and thalidomide (known as MPT). Different drugs and combinations are used for futher relapses; in addition, bisphosphonates may be given to reduce calcium in the blood and lessen the chance of bone fractures and

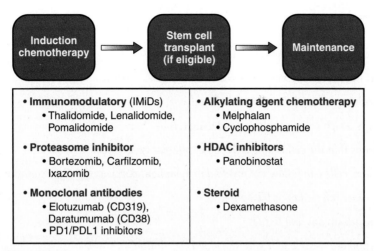

Fig. 2.8 Treatment options for myeloma.

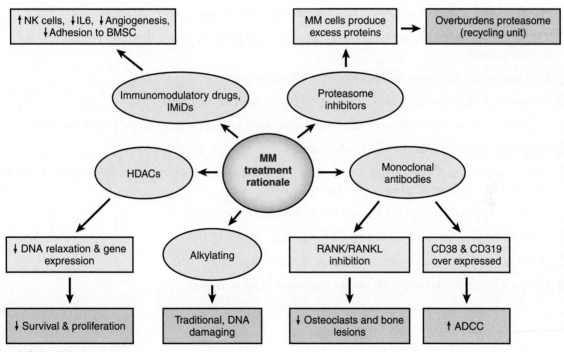

Fig. 2.9 Rationale for treatments.

radiotherapy may be given to locally bony deposits which are causing pain or likely to fracture.

However, myeloma is still considered an incurable disease; with the range of treatment options now available, many will continue to live with the disease for many years, with approximately a third of patients living more than 10 years compared with approximately 5% just 30 years ago.

SELF-ASSESSMENT QUESTIONS

Answer true or false to the following. Answers are on page 165–166.

1   *The circulatory system is synonymous with the cardiovascular system.*

2   *The blood cells make up most of the plasma in blood.*

3   *Red bone marrow is a rich source of blood-producing tissue.*

4   *Pluripotential means that the cell is able to become different types of cells.*

5   *Haematopoietic stem cells can follow the myeloid or lymphoid pathways of differentiation.*

6   *Platelets are otherwise referred to as basophils.*

7   *Lymph drains towards organs and tissues.*

8   *Ultimately, the lymphatic vessels join with the blood circulation.*

9   *Lymph nodes contain lymphocytes.*

10   *Haematopoietic disease manifests in an over-production of one or more types of blood cell.*

11   *Chronic haematopoietic disease is typified by the presence of primitive blast cells in the bone marrow and peripheral blood.*

12   *Myeloid disease results in an over-production of T lymphocytes.*

13   *Chronic myeloid leukaemia is associated with the Philadelphia chromosome.*

14   *Acute myeloid leukaemia is diagnosed by bone marrow aspirate that contains more than 50% blast cells.*

15   *Acute lymphoblastic leukaemia mainly affects adults.*

16   *Chronic lymphocytic leukaemia and non-Hodgkin small lymphocytic lymphoma are recognised by the World Health Organization as the same type of disease.*

17   *Hodgkin lymphoma is typified by the presence of Reed–Sternberg cells.*

18   *Follicular NHL is classified as a high-grade lymphoma.*

19   *Myeloma is characterised by over-proliferation of mature B cells.*

20   *There is no difference between symptomatic and smouldering myeloma.*

Sarcoma

Chapter Outline

Objectives

By the end of this chapter, the reader should be able to:

- Describe the general anatomy of soft tissue and bone.
- Differentiate between sarcoma and carcinoma.
- Outline the characteristics of soft tissue sarcoma and bone sarcoma with reference to specific genetic variants.
- Relate the principles of staging for sarcoma with general treatment strategy.
- Understand the treatment options available for patients with sarcoma.

Sarcoma is the collective term for a group of malignant diseases that originate from connective tissues. Different to epithelial tissue, connective tissue is the packaging material of the body, separating, protecting and supporting various organs (see Chapter 1). All the cells of the connective tissues arise from a layer of tissue found in the early embryo called the mesoderm, the cells of which are called mesenchyme cells (see Chapter 1). This middle layer of the developing embryo differentiates into all types of connective tissues, including cartilage, bone and the connective tissue proper, as well as muscle, blood and the vessels of the blood and lymphatic systems. Mesenchymal cells (a.k.a. pericytes because they are often found around blood vessels) are multipotent; that is, they can differentiate into several cell types as depicted in Fig. 3.1. They are found in abundance in newborns, around 1 in every 10,000 cells, but they decrease in number dramatically to around 1 in every 2 million by 80 years. Mesenchymal cells help regenerate tissue and aid in wound healing, which is why it generally takes longer to recover from injury as the person gets older. This shared origin is perhaps why their oncology and forms of treatment are similar. Each type of connective tissue originates

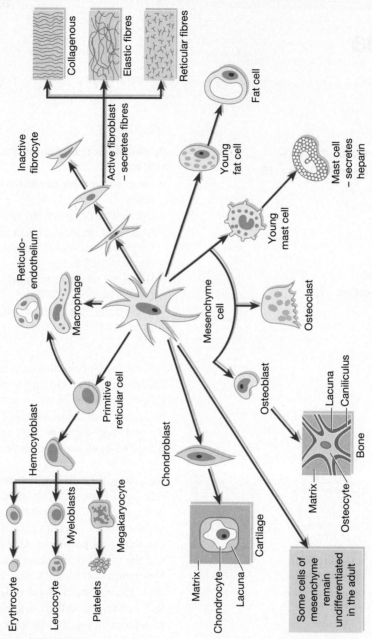

Fig. 3.1 Differentiation of mesenchymal cells.

from an immature type of cell called a blast cell. Blast cells continually reproduce themselves and are found in fibrous tissue (fibroblasts), cartilage (chondroblasts) and bone (osteoblasts). They all produce a matrix that consists of a fluid, semi-fluid, gelatinous or calcified ground substance and protein fibres, the consistency of which depends on the type of cell that produces it. Once the matrix is secreted, the blast cells differentiate into mature cells that are known as fibrocytes, chondrocytes and osteocytes, respectively.

Types of Connective Tissue

Connective tissues can be divided into bone (including cartilage) and soft tissues. Such division is useful when considering the oncology associated with these different types.

CARTILAGE

Cartilage can also be divided into three main types: hyaline cartilage, fibrocartilage and elastic cartilage (Fig. 3.2A).

- Hyaline cartilage is an elastic tissue with a firm matrix filled with groups of cells called chondrocytes that lie in the lacunae. Hyaline cartilage is an earlier more immature form of bone and found as the costal cartilage in ribs, trachea, larynx and bronchi. Hyaline cartilage is also found on the articular surfaces of some bones at synovial joints.
- Fibrocartilage forms a tissue with a mass of white fibres as the matrix, with many fewer chondrocytes than hyaline cartilage. Fibrocartilage is still a strong tissue but has much more elasticity than the hyaline type. It is found in areas of the body that need extra cushioning and protection, such as the disks between vertebrae in the spine.
- Elastic cartilage is a mass of yellow fibres in a matrix with very few chondrocytes; this tissue is found in the pinna (external part of the ear) and epiglottis.

BONE

Bone is one of the hardest tissues of the body and forms the skeleton, which is made up of 206 bones in the adult. The skeleton is the framework of the human body to which all other organs and tissues are attached. The skeleton is divided into two parts: the axial skeleton, composed of the skull, spine and ribs, and the appendicular skeleton (Latin *appendere*: to hang onto), which includes bones of the upper and lower limbs (extremities) plus the shoulder girdle and pelvic girdle.

Bone is covered by a protective, fibrous membrane called the periosteum (Fig. 3.3). The periosteum is composed of two layers: an outer tough fibrous layer that gives strength and an inner thinner layer that provides nourishment via a blood supply and has specialised bone cells called osteoblasts. Osteoblasts are stimulated to produce a protective cuff around a break, so repair can occur from within the bone. Under the periosteum are two further layers: an outer layer of hard, compact bone that provides the supportive strength of the bone and in long bones forms the major part of the shaft (or diaphysis; see Fig. 3.3) and an inner layer of cancellous or spongy bone. Compact bone is made up of closely packed units called osteons or the Haversian system. The osteon is made up of concentric layers called lamellae with spaces between layers called lacunae. In these lacunae lie the bone cells or osteocytes. Cancellous or spongy bone is made of a network whose parts are called trabeculae and give lightness and strength to the bone. The trabeculae provide spaces for red bone marrow and are found at the epiphyses (growth ends) of long bones and in other bones that do not have a medullary cavity (the central space in long bones that is filled with marrow). In a young child, the medullary cavity is full of red marrow, a thick jelly-like substance responsible for blood cell production that is full of red and white blood cells all at different stages of development. As the child matures, this red marrow gradually changes into yellow marrow that no longer produces blood cells. By adulthood, the areas of blood-producing marrow are reduced to the head of the femur, the head of the humerus, the flat bones, and the irregular hip bone. The latter two are common sites for bone marrow biopsy. The proportion of compact to spongy bone varies with different types of bones that can be classified according to their shape – long, short, flat and irregular.

Bone has a number of important roles:

- Support
- Protection
- A 'store' for minerals – calcium and phosphate are released as ions into the bloodstream and later returned to bone; an imbalance in this exchange can exacerbate the condition of osteoporosis in later life.
- Blood cell formation site – haematopoiesis occurs in the red marrow of certain bones.

SOFT TISSUES

Soft tissue can be found around the body and includes tissues such as fat, fibrous, vessels and muscle. Consequently, malignant tumours in this tissue can be found anywhere in the body.

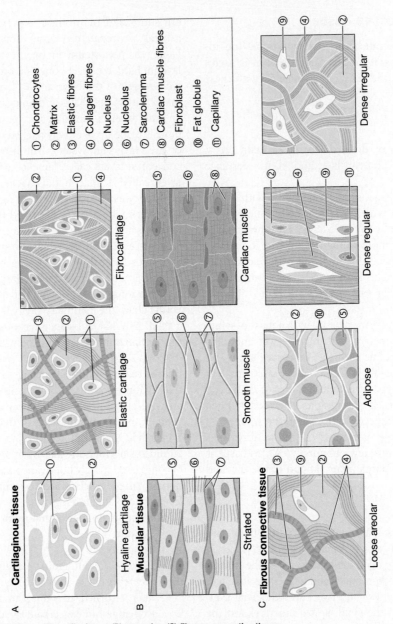

Fig. 3.2 Mature connective tissue: (A) cartilaginous; (B) muscular; (C) fibrous connective tissue.

MUSCLE

There are three main types of muscle tissue: striated muscle, smooth muscle and cardiac muscle (see Fig. 3.2B).

Striated muscle (rhabdomyo-) is under voluntary control. It allows movement, as in the extension and flexion of the upper arm by the presence of two sets of opposing muscle groups: the biceps brachii and triceps. Striated muscle tissue is so called because its appearance under a microscope is of bands of alternating dark and light stripes. Striated muscle cells are cylindrical in shape; there can be more than one nucleus in each cell, and their length can vary from a

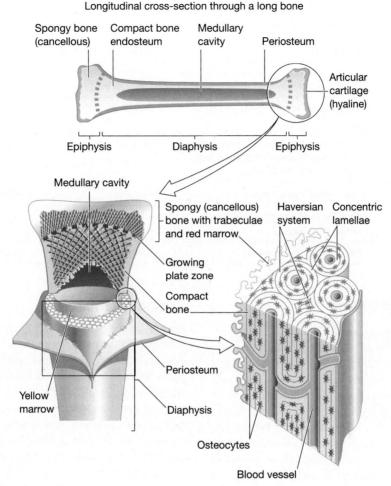

Longitudinal cross-section through a long bone

Spongy bone (cancellous)   Compact bone endosteum   Medullary cavity   Periosteum

Articular cartilage (hyaline)

Epiphysis   Diaphysis   Epiphysis

Medullary cavity

Spongy (cancellous) bone with trabeculae and red marrow

Haversian system   Concentric lamellae

Growing plate zone

Compact bone

Yellow marrow

Periosteum

Diaphysis

Osteocytes

Blood vessel

Fig. 3.3 Anatomy of bone.

few millimetres to over 30 cm. For example, striated muscles can range from small muscles in the front of the neck (suprahyoid and infrahyoid) that aid the act of swallowing to the sartorius muscle, the longest muscle in the body, arising in the pelvis and attached to the medial surface of the tibia of the lower leg. A protective layer called the sarcolemma covers the muscle cell. Striated muscle cells are grouped into bundles and covered by strong white connective tissue called the muscle fascia. Striated muscle is found mainly on the appendicular skeleton.

Smooth (leiomyo-) or involuntary muscle is found in the walls of the gastrointestinal tract, ureters, bladder and blood and lymphatic vessels. These cells are spindle shaped and have one central nucleus. They also form bundles but are held together by sheets of areolar tissue.

Cardiac muscle is only found in the heart and unique in its power of sustained rhythmic contractions.

General Oncology of Connective Tissue

Sarcoma is the term generally used to describe a malignant tumour of connective tissue. However, benign tumours of soft tissue (non-bone connective tissue) are much more common than malignant ones. Benign and malignant tumours of connective tissue are listed in Table 3.1.

TABLE 3.1 Types of Connective Tissue and Associated Benign and Malignant Tumours

Connective Tissue Type	Sites Found	Benign Tumour (-oma)	Malignant Tumour (-sarcoma)
Cartilage	Long bones around knees, pelvis, and hand joints	Chondroma	Chondrosarcoma
Bone	Long bones around knee, shoulder, wrist	Osteoma	Osteosarcoma, Ewing sarcoma
Fat	Surface of shoulders, buttocks, deep in muscles, between the spine and intestine (retroperitoneum)	Lipoma	Liposarcoma
Fibrous tissue	Skin, bone, ovary, breast	Fibroma	Fibrosarcoma
Voluntary muscle	Muscles of appendicular skeleton (arms, legs, etc.)	Rhabdomyoma (rare)	Rhabdomyosarcoma
Involuntary muscle	Skin, stomach, intestines	Leiomyoma	Leiomyosarcoma

SOFT TISSUE SARCOMAS

Soft tissue sarcomas can occur in any part of the body in any connective tissue – muscle, fat, fibrous tissue and blood vessels – giving rise to over 50 subtypes, and they can occur at any age. Most soft tissue sarcomas occur spontaneously with no real known cause, and those that do not are often associated with a genetic mutation; for example, genetic syndromes, such as hereditary retinoblastoma, Li–Fraumeni syndrome and neurofibromatosis, will increase the risk of soft tissue sarcoma. Exposure to radiation, maybe for a previous cancer, can increase the risk of developing sarcomas , as can exposure to certain industrial chemicals, such as PVC and arsenic. Sarcomas tend to occur in a younger age group than do carcinomas.

PRESENTING SYMPTOMS

Patients usually see the doctor because of a painless lump that could have been present for weeks or months. Generally, it is more likely to be malignant if it is deep seated and larger than 5 cm and if the tumour invades local soft tissue, nerves and blood vessels, which leads to early blood-borne spread to the lungs. Lymphatic involvement is uncommon except in the case of synovial sarcoma and alveolar rhabdomyosarcoma. Retroperitoneal sarcomas can grow to a considerable size before giving symptoms, the most common being backache, and movement can become limited if the sarcoma is close to joints.

DIAGNOSIS AND STAGING

Routine investigations to aid diagnosis would include MRI and CT scans to localise the extent of the disease, and multiple core biopsy undertaken by a skilled professional is essential in determining the histological variety of sarcoma. The stage of soft tissue sarcomas and grade are important indicators to determine appropriate treatment, and staging will be modified according to the area of body involved. Extremities, superficial trunk and retroperitoneal masses are based on the size of the mass, as will any head and neck sarcomas, whereas thoracic and abdominal visceral tumours will be based on whether the mass is confined to one or more organs and is solitary or multisited within those areas. Any overall stage will also incorporate the grade of the tumour, and often the French Grading System will be used (Table 3.2).

TREATMENT

Patients with an early stage (stage I) soft tissue sarcoma may be treated with surgery alone if the tumour can be completely resected, including a wide margin of normal tissue. This leaves the patient with a good functional and cosmetic result. However, with inoperable disease, or if enough margin cannot be taken, radiotherapy is administered before surgery, as the tumour is more likely to recur locally. Incomplete excision may be supplemented by radiotherapy. Soft tissue sarcomas

TABLE 3.2 French Grading System for Soft Tissue Sarcomas

French Grading system (FNCLCC)		
Differentiation	Well differentiated	1
	Moderate	2
	Poor	3
Mitotic count	0-9 mitoses	1
	10-19 mitoses	2
	20 or more mitoses	3
Tumour Necrosis	None	1
	Less than or equal to 50%	2
	More than 50%	3

Grade 1 = 2 or 3 (considered Low grade)
Grade 2 = 4 or 5 (considered High grade)
Grade 3 = 6-8 (considered High grade)

are moderately sensitive to chemotherapy, and typically a combination of doxorubicin (Adriamycin) and ifosfamide is used. At stages II and III, a number of patients will have tumours that recur, and although chemotherapy can increase the disease-free interval, it has not affected patients' overall survival.

PROGNOSIS

Treatment outcome tends to be worse with large tumours, deep-seated tumours or high-grade tumours; incomplete excision; and presence of metastases. Patients with early-stage disease have a very good prognosis. Overall, around 70% of people will survive 5 years, with that falling to 20% for late stage.

Notable soft tissue sarcomas include rhabdomyosarcoma and gastrointestinal stromal tumours (GISTs). The general characteristics of other soft tissue sarcomas can be found in Table 3.3.

Rhabdomyosarcoma

Rhabdomyosarcoma differs from other soft tissue sarcomas in that, first, 70% of patients are children (the average

age is 4 years at the time of diagnosis) and, second, when it metastasises, the spread is to bone marrow and lymph nodes. It will present in striated, voluntary muscle, often in the limbs or head and neck region. Li–Fraumeni and hereditary retinoblastoma syndromes increase the risk, and three notable subtypes exist that will have a bearing on disease progression, treatment and outcome. Embryonal rhabdomyosarcoma is the most common subtype and tends to affect children around the head and neck area. Alveolar rhabdomyosarcoma, associated with t(1:13) or t(2:13) genetic abnormalities, often occurs in the limbs, and pleomorphic rhabdomyosarcoma tends to occur more in the limbs of adults.

TREATMENT

Generally, chemotherapy alongside surgery will be the treatment of choice. Chemotherapy will tend to involve a combination of vincristine, Adriamycin (doxorubicin) and cyclophosphamide (VAC), maybe with ifosfamide. The pleomorphic subtype is largely chemoresistant; therefore, radiotherapy alongside surgery will be the treatment of choice.

PROGNOSIS

Embryonal rhabdomyosarcoma is very curable: With current chemotherapy regimens, over 60% of patients are alive and well at 5 years. However, long-term follow-up is required as long-term effects are now being exhibited by these patients. Alveolar rhabdomyosarcoma has a poorer outlook than embryonal, mainly because a large portion will have metastases at presentation. In adults with embryonal rhabdomyosarcoma, although the tumour responds well to the children's chemotherapy regimens, the overall prognosis is much poorer.

GASTROINTESTINAL STROMAL TUMOURS

GISTs can be found throughout the GI tract, mainly in the stomach, the 'stroma' referring to the supporting structures of an organ and, specifically in this case, the muscularis propria. GIST arises from the *Cells of Cajal*, whose function is to facilitate communication between the autonomic nervous system and the smooth muscle of the stomach, thereby promoting contraction when required. Generally, GISTs will affect persons around 60 years of age and tend to present as a large mass, with typical symptoms, including blood in stools or vomit, anaemia, pain, discomfort and maybe signs of metastases.

TABLE 3.3 General Characteristics of Soft Tissue Sarcomas

	Rhabdo-myosarcoma	Leio-myosarcoma	Fibro-sarcoma	Lipo-sarcoma	Angio-sarcoma
Origin	Striated muscle Limbs, H&N	Smooth muscle Uterus, GI, retro	Fibroblasts Often adjacent to bone or deep tissue	Adipocytes (fat cells) Limbs, abdomen	Endothelium of vessels
Aetiology	<5 years Li–Fraumeni Neurofibromatosis	Adults >20 years	Males, 30–40 years	40–60 years, males	PVC, arsenic, lymphoedema previous RT
Pathology	Embryonal (~60%) Alveolar (~20%) t(2:13), t(1:13) Pleomorphic Spindle cell	Pleomorphic	Well (more collagen leads to herringbone pattern) to poorly differentiated	Well differentiated (most common) Myxoid Pleomorphic Dedifferentiated	Early mets haemorrhagic necrotic High grade
Treatment	Surgery Chemo (VAC (I)) RT	Surgery Dox/Ifos Trabectedin	Surgery RT ± CT post surgery	Surgery + RT Trabectedin (Yondelis)	Surgery Dox/Ifos

VAC (I), Vincristine, Adriamycin, Cyclophosphamide (ifosfamide).

Unfortunately, while many patients will present with late-stage disease, early-stage disease may be found incidentally while undergoing investigations for some other ailment.

Staging CT or PET scans can be used to gauge the extent of the mass, and immunohistochemical testing will often indicate mutated cKIT receptor (85% of cases) and/or mutated PGDFR (5% to 10%), with 5% to 10% having wild-type (normal) versions of these.

TREATMENT

Treatment will be determined by whether the disease is localised or advanced and whether or not there is receptor positivity. Surgery in most cases will be the treatment of choice and, if the disease is advanced, treatment with cKIT directed therapies, such as imatinib (Glivec), would be the first-line treatment alongside surgery. PDGFR-positive disease is generally resistant to imatinib, and in such cases the use of this targeted therapy is contraindicated. In such cases, and for those who find imatinib intolerable, second-line treatment, such as the antiangiogenic sunitinib or third-line regorafenib, may be used.

Bone Sarcomas

Primary malignant tumours of bone are very rare, with metastases in the bone and benign tumours such as

TABLE 3.4 Grading for Malignant Bone Tumours

Low Grade	High Grade
• Low cellularity	• High cellularity
• Better/well differentiated	• Poorly differentiated
• Low mitotic count	• High mitotic count
• Low cellular abnormality	• Pleomorphic
• Slow growth, localised	• Rapid growth, invasion and metastasis

osteochondroma, osteoclastoma (giant cell), osteoblastoma and osteoid osteoma being more common. Symptoms will depend on the size and location of the tumour but will typically include a mass or swelling in the affected area and maybe pain, particularly at night. Systemic symptoms of fever, night sweats and weight loss are common. Patients may also present with metastatic disease, often in the lungs, giving rise to dyspnoea.

Typical investigation will include radiography along with a core biopsy carried out at a specialist centre. Blood tests may reveal raised alkaline phosphatase (osteosarcoma) or raised erythrocyte sedimentation rate (Ewing). Furthermore, genetic analysis of the biopsy is important for differential diagnosis (see later).

TABLE 3.5 General Treatment Options for Bone Tumours

Treatment/Type	Osteosarcoma	Chondrosarcoma	Ewing Sarcoma
Surgery	Limb sparing where possible Might need full amputation	Limb sparing where possible Might need full amputation	Post chemotherapy limb sparing
Chemotherapy	Neoadjuvant and adjuvant setting • Doxorubicin • Cisplatin • High-dose methotrexate • Ifosfamide	Rarely	Vincristine Ifosfamide Doxorubicin Etoposide
Radiotherapy	Rarely	Possibly, if incomplete resection	Can be used prior to surgery
Other	Mifamurtide (Mepact) • Immunostimulatory drug • Only in young people (2–30 years)		*Euro-Ewing 99 trial* VIDE + surgery + radiotherapy + busulfan + stem cell transplant

GRADE AND STAGE

Both grade and stage will play an important role. Bone tumour will be graded as low or high grade (Table 3.4), and staging will be influenced by the location of the tumour in the case of the TNM or whether the tumour is confined to the compartment of the bone or not in the case of the Enneking staging system. Both systems will include the grade in the final stage grouping.

TREATMENT

General principles to treatment will consider the likely propensity of these tumours to metastasise and, as such, a combination of limb-sparing surgery with adjunctive chemotherapy, maybe neoadjuvant, will be given. Table 3.5 presents the likely treatment options available.

Notable malignant tumours of bone include osteosarcoma, Ewing sarcoma, and chondrosarcoma.

Osteosarcoma

Osteosarcoma is the most common primary malignant tumour of bone. It arises in the bone-forming cells called osteoblasts. There are two peak age ranges: the first peak appears in adolescence (three-quarters of patients are in this group) between the ages of 10 and 20 years, accounting for about 5% of childhood and adolescent tumours; the second peak appears in the elderly (over 60), often due to a complication of Paget disease or previous radiotherapy. Osteosarcoma is slightly more common in males and typically arises in the metaphysis of long bones, such as the distal femur. In children, over 50% of osteosarcomas arise in the proximal tibia or proximal femur. In the older patient, osteosarcoma can arise in flat as well as long bones. As the tumour enlarges it produces osteoid tissue, forces through the cortex and raises the periosteum. This gives rise to the classic appearance seen on x-ray called Codman triangle, and irradiating spindles of new bone formation gives a typical 'sunburst' appearance. 'Skip' lesions may also occur where tumour cells may not invade immediately adjacent normal tissue but then invade normal tissue some distance away from the primary tumour. It is vital that treatment take this into account, as it will lead to local recurrence.

AETIOLOGY

There is no known cause of osteosarcoma; however, there are a number of genetic mutations that are associated with an increased risk of developing osteosarcomas or sarcomas. Li–Fraumeni syndrome, resulting from a mutation of the p53 tumour suppressor gene, causes the cells to go out of control, leading to an overproduction of cells and the development of sarcomas before the mid-40s, a relatively early age. An increased frequency of osteosarcoma (up to 400-fold) is associated with families with hereditary retinoblastoma (an Rb gene mutation that prevents it from functioning properly as a tumour suppressor gene).

TREATMENT

The mainstay of treatment for osteosarcoma is surgery, which aims to avoid amputation in favour of limb sparing. The use of concurrent chemotherapy has greatly improved survival rates, with typical combination regimens that include doxorubicin and cisplatin. Preoperative chemotherapy has been useful to reduce tumour size and allow previously unsuitable patients to have surgery, and this has increased overall survival rates. For younger patients, the immunomodulatory drug mifamurtide (Mepact) might be used.

PROGNOSIS

With the use of concurrent chemotherapy, overall survival rates of 50% to 80% can be achieved. Up to 20% of patients already have metastases at the time of diagnosis; however, with aggressive chemotherapy, up to 40% of these patients have the chance of long-term survival.

Ewing Sarcoma

Ewing sarcoma is a primary malignant bone tumour that mainly affects children and adolescents, particularly between the ages of 10 and 16 years, and often coincides with periods of rapid bone growth, yet Ewing sarcoma remains rare in all groups of the population. At the time of diagnosis, most patients with Ewing, sarcomas display a change in genetic make-up. A piece of chromosome 11 moves to chromosome 22 and vice versa – a translocation, t(11; 22), where the combination of two unrelated genes creates a new gene that seems to be involved with abnormal control of other genes. This t(11; 22) translocation is unique to Ewing and this genetic change only occurs in the tumour cells, so it is not passed from parent to child or from patients to their progeny. It accounts for 4% of childhood malignancies and affects slightly more males than females; it is rare in Black populations. Ewing sarcoma can arise anywhere in the appendicular skeleton, but the commonest sites are the proximal humerus,

femur and pelvis. Ewing sarcoma typically arises at the diaphysis of the bone, growing subperiosteally; as the tumour enlarges and lays down further bone cells, it can give rise to an 'onion skin' appearance that can be seen on x-ray. The symptoms are very similar to those of other sarcomas and only differ in their sporadic nature; Ewing sarcoma can cause extreme pain.

TREATMENT

Chemotherapy is the mainstay of treatment and has improved the outlook for patients with Ewing sarcoma. Current regimes will follow the Euro-Ewing's 2012 trial protocol that consists of neoadjuvant chemotherapy with vincristine, doxorubicin and cyclophosphamide followed by surgery, if applicable. Further chemotherapy may be given with ifosfamide and etoposide, with Mesna being given to prevent or reduce the effects of ifosfamide on the lining of the bladder. Over 90% of patients already have micrometastases, even though the primary appears localised at the time of diagnosis, and the micrometastases may be undetected by diagnostic tests. Radiotherapy may be given if the tumour is unresectable or only partially resected.

PROGNOSIS

The outlook for patients was very poor until chemotherapy trials in the late 1980s established effective regimens; now, because of these, more than 60% of patients with localised disease are disease free at 5 years. However, if metastases are present, the 5-year survival drops to 20% to 30%.

Chondrosarcoma

Chondrosarcoma is a malignant tumour of cartilage and is the second most common bone tumour after osteosarcoma. Males are twice as likely to develop chondrosarcoma as females, and it rarely develops before the age of 30. The most common sites are the shoulder, pelvis and ribs. There is no known cause; however, there is an association with Paget disease and pre-existing bone disease such as osteochondromas, especially enchondromata (a benign cartilage tumour that, as it grows, stays confined within the metaphysis of long bones). Usually slow-growing, it gives rise to a painful enlarging mass with a wide range of malignancies that are graded from G1 through G4. The majority of tumours are well differentiated with a low risk of metastasis. Most conventional chondrosarcomas are of low grade, but aggressive forms, such as de-differentiated and mesenchymal varieties, may present, but these are very rare.

TREATMENT

Surgery is the treatment of choice, if the tumour is well to moderately differentiated. Generally, these tumours are not responsive to chemotherapy, but this may be used if the tumour is of an aggressive nature or metastases are present. Likewise, radiotherapy is largely ineffective but may be used if the tumour is unresectable.

PROGNOSIS

Prognosis is very much dependent on the location of the tumour, the grade and whether metastases are present.

Well to moderately differentiated tumours tend to metastasise very late, if at all, and consequently have a good prognosis, with around 80% to 90% of patients surviving 5 years or more. Poorly differentiated tumours tend to metastasise early, and the prognosis is much poorer.

Point to note – treatment of sarcomas tends to involve high-dose chemotherapy alongside aggressive surgery. Young people will experience long-term side effects to treatment, such as orthopaedic issues and long-term fatigue, and there may be problems with kidney and hormone function, with infertility a real risk when using such chemotherapy drugs. The possibility of secondary cancer must also be carefully monitored as well as cardiac toxicity, as anthracycline chemotherapy drugs are often used as part of the treatment regimen.

SELF-ASSESSMENT QUESTIONS

Answer true or false to the following. Answers are on page 165–166.

1. Every type of connective tissue derives from an immature type of cell called a blast cell.
2. The protective fibrous outer layer of the bone is called the cortex.
3. Chondrocytes are groups of cells found in cartilage.
4. Striated muscle is not under voluntary control.
5. Sarcoma is the collective term for all types of connective tissue tumours.
6. The most common connective tissue tumour in children is Ewing sarcoma.
7. The majority of sarcomas arise spontaneously.
8. Sarcomas in general present with a painful lump.
9. Osteosarcoma is more common in young people.
10. The classic appearance of osteosarcoma on x-ray is called the Codman triangle.
11. Ewing sarcoma more commonly arises in the appendicular skeleton.
12. In most cases of Ewing sarcoma, there is a specific genetic mutation: the chromosome translocation t(11;22).
13. Surgery is the treatment of choice for Ewing sarcoma.
14. In chondrosarcoma, the shoulder, pelvis and ribs are the most common sites.
15. The majority of chondrosarcomas are of low grade and have a low risk of metastasis.
16. In Ewing sarcoma, the older the child, the better the prognosis.
17. Radiotherapy is the main treatment of choice for soft tissue sarcomas.
18. Embryonal rhabdomyosarcoma has the best prognosis of the sarcomas.
19. GIST is often associated with mutated BRaf.
20. Imatinib is often used to treat advanced GIST.

The Nervous System – Brain Tumours

Objectives

By the end of this chapter, the reader should be able to:

- Differentiate between the functions of neurons and glial cells.
- Explain the anatomic location and functions of the cerebrum, brain stem, cerebellum, spinal cord, peripheral nerves and cerebrospinal fluid.
- Differentiate between the most common types of brain tumours.
- Understand grading of brain tumour with reference to glioblastoma.
- Explain the role of surgery, chemotherapy and radiotherapy in the treatment of brain tumours.

The nervous system is the control system of the body, carrying out many activities that can be divided into sensory, integrative and motor functions. We are able to sense external and internal stimuli, interpret the changes sensed, and respond to this change by muscular contraction or glandular secretion. The nervous system, along with the endocrine system, maintains homeostasis within the body; in other words, these two systems keep the internal environment constant.

The various subdivisions of the nervous system can be seen in Fig. 4.1, the principal division being between the central nervous system (CNS) and the peripheral nervous system (PNS). The PNS incorporates an afferent pathway conveying information to the CNS and an efferent pathway conveying information away from the CNS. Furthermore, the efferent pathway is divided into the somatic and autonomic pathways. The somatic pathway carries nerve impulses to skeletal muscle, which is under conscious control and produces voluntary movement, whereas the autonomic pathway carries impulses to smooth muscle, glands and cardiac muscle, which are not under conscious control and therefore move involuntarily.

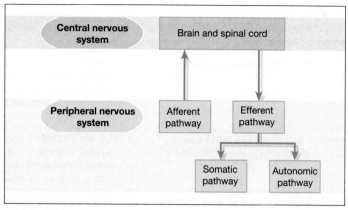

Fig. 4.1 Subdivisions of the nervous system.

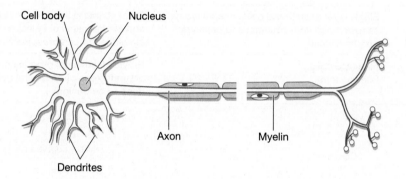

Fig. 4.2 A neuron.

The nervous system consists of only two types of cells: neurons (nerve cells) and neuroglia (glial cells that support the neurons). Neurons are cells that carry messages through the body by electrochemical processes, and they differ from other cells in the body in that they have specialised extensions called dendrites and axons (Fig. 4.2), which bring information to and from the cell body, respectively.

Axons may be covered by a myelin sheath, which insulates the axon and increases nerve impulse speed. Neurons, after about 6 months of age, lose the mitotic apparatus enabling cell division to occur, which means that nerve cells have a limited ability to regenerate and renew themselves. As a result, many are never replaced when they die; consequently, the number of nerve cells is reduced as the body ages. It is rare, therefore, to develop malignant tumours of neurons. The vast majority of malignant tumours of the CNS are of the supporting glial cells.

In the PNS, there may be some repair of damage because different supporting cells are responsible for the myelination in the two systems. In the PNS, myelination of axons is performed by neurolemmocytes or Schwann cells, which proliferate after damage to the axon. In the CNS, myelination is performed by oligodendrocytes, which do not survive after damage to the axon. Myelin gives a white appearance to brain tissue, and unmyelinated axons appear grey; hence the terms white and grey matter when referring to tissues of the CNS.

Glial cells have many important functions without which neurons would not work (Table 4.1).

The Central Nervous System

THE BRAIN

The brain is composed of the cerebrum, cerebellum, diencephalon and brain stem, the lower end of which is continuous with the spinal cord (Fig. 4.3).

TABLE 4.1	Supporting Cells of the Nervous System	
Cell Type	**Description Tumour Type**	**Function**
Astrocyte	Star-shaped cells with many projections Astrocytoma (astro = star)	Provide neurons with physical and nutritional support; clean up debris; transport nutrients; hold neurons in place; digest parts of dead neurons; and regulate the content of extracellular space
Oligodendrocytes	Similar to astrocytes but with fewer Oligodendroglioma projections (oligo = few)	Provide insulation; provide support by semirigid connective tissue between neurons and produce myelin sheath around axons of central nervous system
Microglia	Small cells (micro) also referred to as microglioma brain macrophages because they destroy dead cells and microbes	Digest parts of dead cells and destroy microbes
Ependyma	Single layer of epithelial cells; ependymoma shapes range from squamous to columnar; may be ciliated	Form epithelial lining for ventricles of brain and central canal of spinal cord. Related to circulation of cerebrospinal fluid
Schwann cells	Flattened cells Schwannoma	Provide insulation; produce myelin sheath around axons of peripheral nervous system (tend to be benign)

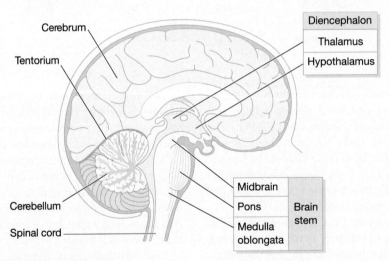

Fig. 4.3 Principal parts of the brain in sagittal section.

The cerebrum, the largest component of the brain, is composed of the right and left cerebral hemispheres. An outer layer of grey matter, the cerebral cortex, is arranged in a number of folds called gyri or convolutions. The deep grooves that occur between these folds are called fissures or sulci, the largest of which, the longitudinal fissure, incompletely separates the two hemispheres. Below this fissure, the two hemispheres are connected by the corpus callosum, which is a large bundle of nerve fibres. Each hemisphere is divided

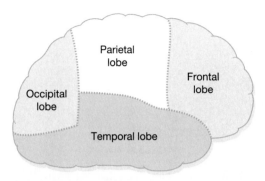

Fig. 4.4 The lobes of the brain.

TABLE 4.2	The Functions of the Lobes of the Brain
Lobe	**Function**
Frontal	Attention, thought, reasoning, behaviour, movement, smell and sexual urges
Parietal	Intellect, reasoning, touch, internal stimuli, language, reading and visual functions
Temporal	Behavior, memory, hearing, visual functions and emotions
Occipital	Vision

descriptively into four lobes (Fig. 4.4) – frontal, parietal, temporal and occipital lobes – that derive their names from the cranial bones which cover them.

The different areas of the cerebral cortex have different functions (Table 4.2), which account for varied tumour symptoms, depending on the area involved. Symptoms will also depend on which side of the brain is involved as each side appears to be more important for some functions than others. The right hemisphere is more important for left hand control, sight, touch, taste, smell and sound, whereas the left hemisphere is more important for right hand control, reasoning, language and numerical skills.

The cerebellum, the second largest component of the brain, lies below the occipital lobes of the cerebrum. Like the cerebrum, it is divided into two hemispheres, each containing different lobes separated by fissures. The functions of the cerebellum relate to balance and subconscious skeletal muscle movements, allowing the body to perform well-coordinated movements. The cerebellum is linked to the balance system of the inner ear to maintain equilibrium. A tumour in the cerebellum may result in symptoms relating to lack of balance and uncoordinated movement but, unlike the cerebral hemispheres, the symptoms affect the same side of the body as the damaged lobe.

The diencephalon is composed of the thalamus and hypothalamus, which interpret sensations such as touch, pressure, pain and temperature. The hypothalamus monitors the body's internal environment, including blood temperature and hormone and fluid levels. It also controls the autonomic nervous system and is the link between the nervous and endocrine systems, maintaining homeostasis.

The brain stem is composed of the midbrain, pons, and medulla oblongata. The midbrain connects the cerebral hemispheres. Posteriorly, the midbrain has four rounded eminences that are the reflex centres for sight and hearing. Below this lies the pons, which is composed mainly of nerve fibres passing between the cerebral hemispheres and also between the cerebral hemispheres and the spinal cord. Anatomically, the medulla oblongata is the inferior part of the brain and connects the brain to the spinal cord. In the medulla oblongata, nerve fibres from the cerebrum cross, which accounts for the fact that symptoms of disease can occur on the side of the body opposite that of the brain affected. This is known as the split-brain concept. The other functions of the medulla oblongata are related to consciousness and arousal as well as the vital reflex centres for respiratory, cardiac, and vasomotor functions.

For protection, the brain and spinal cord are covered by three membranes called meninges (Fig. 4.5). Cranial dura mater has two layers: an outer layer that adheres to the cranium (bone) and is known as the periosteal layer and an inner layer known as the meningeal layer.

The cerebellum and cerebrum are separated by a fold of dura mater called the tentorium cerebelli (see Fig. 4.3). This tentorium is an anatomical division useful in distinguishing between the malignant pathologies of the CNS. Supratentorial tumours are confined to the cerebrum, and infratentorial tumours arise in

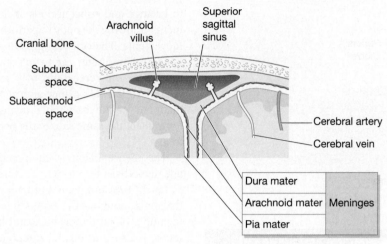

Fig. 4.5 The meninges of the brain.

the cerebellum or brain stem. The pia mater covers the brain, and the arachnoid mater between the dura mater and pia mater contains blood vessels. Further protection is afforded by cerebrospinal fluid (CSF), a clear, colourless fluid secreted by a vascular fold of pia mater called the choroid plexus, which fills the subarachnoid space and bathes the spinal cord (Fig. 4.6). CSF also has a circulatory function, transporting nutrients from the blood to the brain and spinal cord and excreting waste products from the brain and spinal cord to the blood. The flow of CSF around the brain and spinal cord allows metastatic cells from tumours within the CNS to circulate throughout the system, which means that treatment may have to include the entire cerebrospinal axis.

The blood supply to the brain is vital for it to function. Oxygen and glucose, in particular, are vital to cell survival, and these pass quickly from the capillaries to the brain cells. Other substances in the blood do not enter as quickly, and some – for example, proteins and some drugs – do not enter at all because the capillaries of the brain are different in structure from those in the rest of the body. The cells are densely packed and have large numbers of glial cells surrounding them. This is known as the blood–brain barrier. The blood–brain barrier is useful in preventing harmful substances from entering the brain, but this also means that chemotherapy drugs are not always an effective method of treatment, as not all drugs will get through this barrier.

THE SPINAL CORD

The spinal cord lies in the upper two-thirds of the vertebral canal, extending from the upper border of the first cervical vertebra to the lower border of the first lumbar vertebra. The spinal cord is about 43 cm long in women and 45 cm long in men and protected by the vertebral column. Nerves arise in pairs from a series of segments of the spinal cord that are named according to the vertebrae from which they arise. There are 31 pairs in total: 8 cervical, 12 thoracic, 5 lumbar, 5 sacral and 1 coccygeal. Since the spinal cord stops at the first lumbar vertebra, nerves that branch from the cord into lumbar and sacral levels run in the vertebral canal for some distance before they exit. This area is known as the cauda equina, where the nerves that supply the lower part of the body originate higher in the spinal cord, giving rise to symptoms at a distance from an area that is damaged or diseased. For example, the nerves controlling the muscles of the thigh originate at the second lumbar vertebra.

Oncology

Primary CNS tumours are uncommon, accounting for 1% to 2% of all cancers worldwide each year. The overall male:female ratio is 1.5:1, with the vast majority of tumours arising in the brain. A bimodal pattern of incidence with age (with peaks under 10 years and at 55 to 80 years) occurs in CNS tumours.

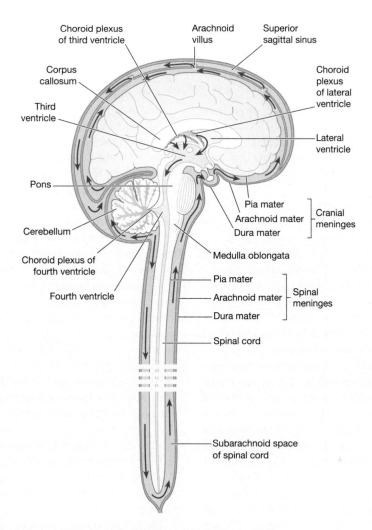

Fig. 4.6 The brain, spinal cord and meninges, with flow of cerebrospinal fluid indicated by *arrows*.

The majority of adults develop supratentorial tumours, whereas the majority of tumours in children are infratentorial. At least one-third of all tumours are secondary or metastatic deposits from other primary sites, including breast and bronchus tumours.

The aetiology of brain tumours is generally unknown, although causative factors may include ionising radiation, occupational carcinogens, petrochemicals, agricultural work and exposure to the rubber industry.

The primary histological types are not of neurons but supporting tissues and glands. Tumours arising from neurons are extremely rare. Eighty-five percent of primary tumours are gliomas arising from a malignant change in mature glial cells. These are named according to the glial cell type affected (see Table 4.1) and include astrocytomas, ependymomas, oligodendrogliomas and medulloblastomas.

Astrocytomas are the most common histological type and arise from astrocytes, a type of supporting cell in the brain. They can be *focal* with a distinct edge (more common in children) or more commonly grow by direct extension into surrounding tissue and are described as *diffuse*. Astrocytomas tend to be classified according to features such as cellular pleomorphism (different cell shapes), mitotic activity (the number of cells undergoing cell division), microvascular proliferation (increase in the number of blood vessels) and necrosis (cell death).

Grade 1 is the least malignant, has none of these features and is referred to as *pilocytic* because it produces a hair-like structure around the cells. Such tumours are very slow-growing and contained and will often occur in the cerebellum of children and young adults.

Grade 2 or 'diffuse' astrocytoma is still referred to as low grade. It tends to have less well-defined edges, and although slow-growing, it may return after surgery as grade 3. It tends to be more common in males between 20 and 45 years of age.

Grade 3 or anaplastic astrocytoma is high grade and poorly differentiated with rapidly dividing cells and will often recur after treatment as grade 4. Again, it is more common in males and affects people between 30 and 70 years of age.

Grade 4 – Often referred to as glioblastoma or glioblastoma multiforme (GBM). A very aggressive, fast-growing, undifferentiated tumour with rapid disease progression and poor survival. Typically, this tumour has a great ability to produce new blood vessels and as such is usually very vascular but also demonstrates areas of necrosis. Glioblastoma can be described as 'primary' or de novo (most common), which develop spontaneously, or *secondary*, which develop from existing lower grade astrocytomas. Primary glioblastoma is now analogous to glioblastoma with isocitrate dehydrogenase (IDH) wild-type (see section later on biomarkers), and secondary GBMs are analogous to astrocytoma IDH mutant (grade 4).

Low-grade astrocytomas are commonly found in the frontal, parietal and temporal lobes of adults and the brain stem and cerebellum of children. Astrocytomas can occur supra- or infratentorial. A biopsy will not always give a clear histological diagnosis of the whole tumour, as mixed varieties are common. If the tumour is highly malignant, it may be impossible to recognise the initial cell of origin. Initially, malignant tumours invade the white matter and then the grey matter, although spread throughout the CNS is rare.

Ependymomas account for 5% of all intracranial tumours and occur mainly in childhood and early adulthood. They are derived from the ciliated lining cells of the CNS cavities, which aid in the circulation of CSF and therefore commonly spread by seeding throughout the CNS via the CSF. Over half arise from infratentorial sites, the most common site for childhood brain tumours. There are essentially three grades of ependymoma. Grade 1 consists of myxopapillary ependymoma, which may occur in the lower part of the spinal column, and subependymoma, which may occur near a ventricle; both are very uncommon, especially in children. Grade 2 is the most common type and simply referred to as ependymoma. The highest grade, grade 3, is anaplastic ependymoma, which, as the name suggests, has more rapid growth.

Oligodendrogliomas, which are derived from oligodendrocytes, typically arise supratentorial in the frontal, parietal, or temporal lobes. They are the third most common type of glioma, more common in adults, and usually have a long indolent history. Oligodendrogliomas are characterised by IDH and 1p/19q codeletions (see biomarker section), which will inform treatment strategy and possible long-term outcome. Typically, these tumours will be grade 2 or 3, with grade 3 tumours being more aggressive and difficult to cure. Characteristic deposits of calcium can be seen on a radiograph and aid in differential diagnosis. When spread via the CSF occurs, it is usually associated with a rapidly growing and occasionally fatal tumour.

Medulloblastomas are derived from the foetal external layer of the cerebellum that does not normally remain in the body after birth and is the most common brain tumour in children. They mainly arise in the cerebellum and often metastasise via the CSF to the spinal cord or other parts of the brain. Occasionally (fewer than 10% of cases) there can be extra neural metastases. Four distinct variants termed WNT, Sonic Hedgehog (SHH), Group 3 and Group 4 exist, and further exploration of these categories might lead to a more targeted approach to treatments in the future. For example, patients with the WNT variety have an excellent prognosis, whereas group 3 patients are more likely to experience CSF seeding and therefore have a poor prognosis. A known risk factor for the SHH subtype is the nevoid basal cell carcinoma syndrome

(NBCCS) – Gorlin syndrome. Early identification of these patients could lead to earlier diagnosis and more successful treatments.

Brain tumours are classified on the basis of tumour cell type, histological grade and molecular and biological markers. For some tumours, location and metastatic spread within the CSF are also used in classification. There is no tumour–node–metastasis (TNM) staging system for CNS tumours.

Spread of Intracranial Tumours

Primary tumours of the CNS spread by local invasion. Metastatic spread outside the CNS is a rare occurrence, mainly, it is thought, because of the lack of lymphatic drainage. Another reason may be that symptoms in this enclosed system tend to present early before spread outside has occurred. Metastatic spread outside the CNS is possible, however, via the CSF if ventriculoperitoneal shunting has been performed to relieve hydrocephalus. Seeding of cells via the CSF can result in multiple deposits on the surface of the brain and spinal cord. This is typical of medulloblastoma, ependymoma and pineoblastoma, which means that treatment has to include the entire cerebrospinal axis.

On the other hand, metastatic spread to the CNS from other sites in the body, such as tumours of the breast and bronchus, occurs commonly. These tumour cells appear to be able to cross the blood–brain barrier. However, this difference could be explained by the fact that primary brain tumours become symptomatic before cells cross the blood–brain barrier rather than in terms of greater permeability to one malignant cell type than another.

Spinal Tumours

Spinal tumours are classified by their site of origin within the meninges (see Fig. 4.6) as extradural, intradural or intramedullary. Extramedullary tumours tend to be metastatic disease, intradural tumours include meningiomas and neurofibromas, and intramedullary tumours include astrocytomas, ependymomas and hemangioblastomas. Tumours often present with symptoms of spinal cord compression, which is seen when the lesion lies between the foramen magnum and the lower limit of the cord or cauda equina compression when the lesion is below the limit of the spinal cord and affects only nerve roots. As mentioned

TABLE 4.3   Clinical Features of Tumours of the Central Nervous System

Cause of Clinical Feature	Description of Clinical Feature
Increased intracranial pressure	Headache, vomiting, papilledema, drowsiness, mental deterioration and personality changes
Cerebellar tumour	Loss of coordination of movement; headaches and vomiting
Frontal lobe tumour	Intellectual impairment and personality change; weakness and paralysis
Temporal lobe tumour	Epilepsy, speech disturbance and visual field defects
Parietal lobe tumour	Sensory or visual inattention, difficulty with writing and simple mathematics
Occipital lobe tumour	Visual field defects, hallucinations and seizures
Brain stem tumour	Cranial nerve defects, involvement of motor and sensory tracts

earlier, spinal nerves emerge from the spinal cord higher than the area they supply; therefore, symptoms of spinal cord compression can include lower limb paralysis.

Clinical Features

Clinical features can arise either from pressure caused by the tumour or from the location of the tumour within the CNS. As mentioned earlier, signs and symptoms will be related to the functions of different areas of the brain (Table 4.3).

Investigations

Investigations for CNS tumours include contrast-enhanced computed tomography (CT) and magnetic resonance imaging (MRI) scans; stereotactic, percutaneous needle biopsy or open biopsy and lumbar puncture for cerebral tumours; and myelogram and open biopsy for spinal tumours. Positron emission tomography (PET) scans combined with CT can be used to assess the extent of the tumour and also check for possible progression of disease after treatment.

Biomarkers

Some brain tumours may demonstrate specific genetic aberrations which, if detected, can help with diagnosis, aggressiveness of the tumour and possible response to treatment.

MGMT test – the *MGMT* (O^6-methylguanine-DNA methyltransferase) gene is responsible for producing the MGMT protein that repairs damaged DNA. Chemotherapy drugs, like temozolomide, an alkylating agent, are often used to treat gliomas. The damage to DNA can be repaired if much of the MGMT protein is present. Methylated *MGMT* genes in tumour cells effectively turn off the action of the MGMT gene, meaning there is less of the MGMT protein present in the tumour microenvironment, leading to a lowered ability to repair DNA following damage from alkylating chemotherapy agents. Testing for methylated *MGMT* genes may therefore be a predictor as to how effective such chemotherapy might be.

1p/19q test – This test may be used to help predict long-term survival in patients with oligodendroglioma (mainly). Sections of genes on chromosomes 1 and 19, respectively, are referred to as 'p' and 'q'. These genes are associated with chemotherapy drug resistance, and if they are absent (deleted), then it may be an indicator that chemotherapy will be more effective, leading to better long-term survival in these patients.

IDH1 and IDH2 tests – Testing for mutations in the *IDH1* and *IDH2* genes is useful in diagnosing certain types of glioma. It is specifically used to aid in the diagnosis of astrocytoma (grade 2 and 3), oligodendroglioma and secondary glioblastoma (see earlier section on astrocytoma).

ATRX and TP53 tests – Mutations in these markers are useful in the differential diagnosis of grade 2/3 glioma and astrocytomas. Tumours that are IDH-mutated, along with mutations in ATRX and TP53, tend to grow more slowly than tumours without the IDH mutation. However, these slow-growing tumours will also be more resistant to radiotherapy.

BRAF test – BRAF is an intercellular signalling protein responsible for the transmission of cell survival and proliferation signals through the MAPK signalling pathway. Mutation of these proteins effectively means the cancer cell receives constant messages to grow and proliferate, leading to tumour development. It is a useful test in diagnosing grade 1 (pilocytic) astrocytoma.

TERT test – Telomerase reverse transcriptase (TERT) plays an essential role in survival and possible immortality of cancer cells. Mutant TERT in cancer cells can lead to prolonged survival of the cancer cells and endless replicative potential. When found with 1p/19q deletions and mutant IDH, it would confirm a diagnosis of oligodendroglioma and may also predict better response to therapy and prolonged survival. If found alone, then survival is usually poorer. TERT found with wild-type (normal) IDH is likely to confirm glioblastoma.

Treatment

Treating tumours within the brain offers its own challenges. Firstly, the brain is susceptible to damage from conventional treatments. Surgery, in particular, will often involve removal of only part of the tumour, as removing too much brain tissue will in itself cause problems. Secondly, the brain, and nervous tissue in general, has limited capacity to repair itself from the damage caused by surgery and radiotherapy. Thirdly, most gliomas are resistant to conventional therapies, and many gliomas will return even after treatment and usually return at a higher grade, with greater infiltration and aggressiveness. And fourthly, many of our chemotherapy drugs will not cross the blood–brain barrier, meaning delivering a tumouricidal dose of chemotherapy is often very difficult.

Generally, management of CNS tumours depends on the location of the tumour, its grade and whether there is spread throughout the system via the CSF. Surgery is recommended for most primary intracranial and spinal tumours if the lesion is accessible without causing neurological problems, and in cases where there is no evidence of seeding throughout the CNS, surgery may be followed by radiotherapy to the tumour bed or residual tumour only. Where there is evidence or the likelihood of seeding via the CSF, such as in medulloblastoma and ependymoma, the entire CNS will require treatment. Steroids, such as dexamethasone, may be given to relieve the effects of raised intracranial pressure.

Patients with grade 1 tumours will usually have their tumour surgically removed, or if they are deemed to be very slow-growing, they may even just be monitored – for example, pilocytic astrocytoma – as often, removal will cause more problems than it solves.

Those with grade 2 tumour will generally be offered surgery, which will often involve only partial removal of the tumour followed by radiotherapy to the tumour bed. Where chemotherapy is deemed suitable, this may be in the form of Gliadel wafers, which are a fibre mesh coated with the chemotherapy drug carmustine. Such an approach circumvents the blood–brain barrier and allows the chemotherapy drug to soak into the area directly where the tumour was.

Further chemotherapy may be offered using temozolomide, but this will depend on the MGMT status as described earlier. PCV (procarbazine, CCNU (lomustine), vincristine) chemotherapy might be used alongside radiotherapy. It has been shown to extend survival, particularly in patients with oligodendroglioma that exhibits 1p/19q codeletions.

Patients with grade 3 and 4 disease offer further challenges as these tumours will be more infiltrative (diffuse) in nature, making total resection impossible in most cases. In both cases, a combination of surgery, radiotherapy, and chemotherapy is common. In the case of grade 4 (glioblastoma), the presence or absence of certain biomarkers (as described earlier) will help in the treatment decision-making process.

After treatment, patients will undergo regular scans to monitor its effectiveness and look for sign of recurrence. Unfortunately, many gliomas will recur after treatment, usually transforming to a higher grade with more diffuse disease. In such cases, further surgery may be offered.

Prognosis

The prognosis of tumours of the CNS depends on their grade, histological type, and extent. Low-grade astrocytomas have the best survival. Around 40% people with grade 2 astrocytomas will survive for 5 years, but this drops to less than 10% for grade IV. Children with low grade gliomas will have a much better survival of around 90% surviving more than 5 years. Similar trends can be seen in other histological types.

SELF-ASSESSMENT QUESTIONS

Answer true or false to the following. Answers are on page 165–166.

1 The CNS comprises the brain and spinal cord.

2 Neurons can renew themselves indefinitely.

3 Glial cells are the supporting cells of the CNS.

4 Oligodendrocytes are responsible for the myelin sheath on peripheral nerves.

5 The cerebellum is the largest component of the brain.

6 The occipital lobe is concerned with balance.

7 Astrocytes are the most abundant glial cell.

8 Primary tumours of the CNS are uncommon.

9 Astrocytoma is the most common histology of primary CNS tumours.

10 Grade 4 astrocytoma and glioblastoma are the same.

11 High levels of MGMT protein mean temozolomide will be more effective.

12 Oligodendrogliomas are characterised by IDH and 1p/19q codeletions.

13 Ependymomas are derived from ciliated lining cells of CNS cavities.

14 *Medulloblastoma is the most common CNS tumour in children.*

15 *SHH is a variety of oligodendroglioma.*

16 *Spread outside the CNS from a brain primary is common.*

17 *Signs and symptoms depend on the site of the tumour.*

18 *Metastatic disease to the brain is common.*

19 *PCV (procarbazine, CCNU (lomustine), vincristine) is a common chemotherapy regimen given post-surgery.*

20 *Prognosis is dependent on the grade of the tumour.*

The Endocrine System

Chapter Outline

Objectives

By the end of this chapter, the reader should be able to:

- Identify the key endocrine glands in the body and the hormones that they release.
- Explain the signs and symptoms associated with tumours of the endocrine system.
- Differentiate between the types of pituitary gland tumours.
- Explain the treatment options available for malignant thyroid tumours.
- Understand the role of surgery, radiotherapy and chemotherapy in the treatment of endocrine tumours.

Two regulatory systems, the nervous system and the endocrine system, work together to maintain equilibrium (homeostasis) of bodily functions. The endocrine system is made up of a series of glands (Fig. 5.1) that secrete hormones directly into the bloodstream to be dispersed throughout the body. This makes them different from exocrine glands that secrete their products into ducts, which in turn transfer them to a body cavity. Hormones are designed to target many different areas of the body. Generally, hormones affect the metabolic rate of cells – that is, how quickly or slowly they break down or re-form the chemicals necessary for cellular survival.

The endocrine glands to be covered in this chapter include the pituitary gland, thyroid gland and adrenal glands. Other organs of the body, such as the small intestine, pancreas, testes and ovary, also contain endocrine tissue. The endocrine functions of these organs are covered in other chapters.

The Pituitary Gland (Hypophysis)

The pituitary gland lies centrally within the sella turcica of the skull in a protected position (Fig. 5.2).

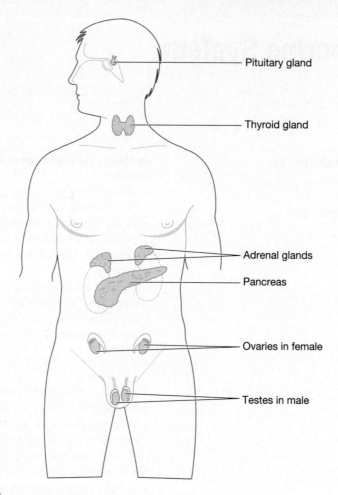

Fig. 5.1 The endocrine system.

The deepest part of the sella turcica is often referred to as the pituitary fossa since the pituitary gland sits in it. The gland is connected to the base of the brain via a stalk called the infundibulum.

Immediately superior to the pituitary gland lies the optic chiasma, where the optic nerves cross. This area can be related to common presenting symptoms for pituitary tumours (see below). The pituitary is composed of an anterior lobe, which is glandular tissue and is sometimes referred to as the adenohypophysis, and a posterior lobe, which is nervous tissue and is referred to as the neurohypophysis.

Microscopically, the anterior pituitary is made up of cells named according to the type of hormone they produce and maybe also according to their affinity for certain staining techniques. The posterior pituitary is a storage area for hormones produced in the hypothalamus. Two hormones are released from the posterior pituitary gland: antidiuretic hormone and oxytocin. Table 5.1 lists the hormones which are produced by these cells and their principal target organs.

ONCOLOGY

Virtually all tumours of the pituitary gland arise from the anterior lobe. They are generally characterised as 'functioning', hormone producing or 'nonfunctioning'. They are invariably benign and curable. Pituitary adenomas present a danger to the individual mainly because of the proximity to vital structures. Any of the tumours may enlarge the sella turcica, causing pressure

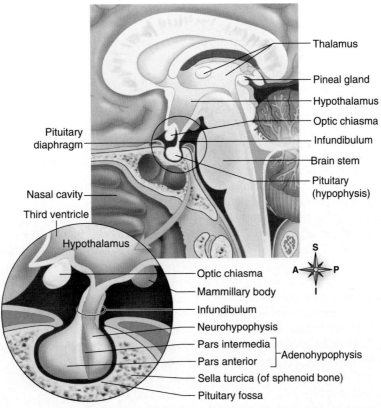

Fig. 5.2 Position of the pituitary gland in the sella turcica. (From Thibodeau GA, Patton KT. *Anatomy and Physiology*. 7th ed. St. Louis, MO: Elsevier; 2009).

TABLE 5.1	**Pituitary Cells, Hormones and Their Target Organs**			
	Stain	**Type of Cell Producing Hormone**	**Hormone**	**Target Organ**
Anterior	Acidophilic	Somatotroph	Growth hormone	General; promotes growth of bone and muscle
		Mammotrophs	Prolactin	Breast
	Basophilic	Corticotrophs	Adrenocorticotrophic hormone (ACTH)	Adrenal cortex
			Melanocyte-stimulating hormone	Skin (melanocytes)
		Thyrotrophs	Thyroid-stimulating hormone (TSH)	Thyroid gland
		Gonadotrophs	Follicle-stimulating hormone (FSH) and luteinising hormone (LH)	Ovaries and testes
Posterior	Neurosecretory		Antidiuretic hormone	Kidneys
			Oxytocin	Uterus

symptoms. Pressure on the optic chiasma causes visual defects, and pressure on the brain may even cause death. Clinical syndromes may also be present with hormonally active tumours. Eosinophilic tumours often secrete growth hormone, resulting in gigantism in younger patients and acromegaly in others. Basophilic tumours secrete prolactin and adrenocorticotropic hormone, resulting in Cushing syndrome.

STAGING

Although generally there is no TNM staging scheme for pituitary adenomas, they will often be classified according to their cell type (see Table 5.1) and size and, in particular, as to whether the adenoma is confined to or invaded beyond the sella turcica.

TREATMENT

Most people suspected of a pituitary gland tumour will be referred to an endocrinologist, particularly if there is evidence of hormonal overactivity. Magnetic resonance and other imaging techniques play an important role in localising and assessing the size and extent of these tumours. The mainstay of treatment is trans-sphenoidal surgery, particularly for those tumours confined to the sella turcica. Any extension beyond the sella turcica may be an indication for external beam radiotherapy. For tumours which secrete excess growth hormone or prolactin, bromocriptine or cabergoline has been successful as a medical treatment. These dopamine antagonists are designed to reduce the amount of growth hormone produced by the tumour by interreacting with the dopamine receptors on the tumour cell surface, which in turn send a message to the cell which inhibits secretion of the hormone.

The Thyroid Gland

The thyroid gland is located just below the larynx (Fig. 5.3). The thyroid consists of a right lobe and left lobe either side of the trachea, joined by a mass of tissue on the anterior aspect of the trachea called the isthmus. Histologically, the thyroid is composed of spherical sacs called thyroid follicles, and the walls of each follicle consist of two types of cells: follicular and parafollicular (C) cells. The follicular cells produce two hormones, thyroxine (T4) and triiodothyronine (T3).

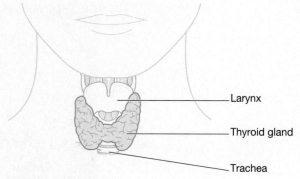

Fig. 5.3 The thyroid gland.

These hormones help regulate metabolism and the process of growth and tissue differentiation. The parafollicular cells secrete calcitonin, a hormone which helps regulate the amount of calcium and phosphates in the blood. The thyroid has a very rich blood supply and is relatively close to the carotid artery. Lymphatic drainage is primarily to the cervical lymph nodes and the pre- and paratracheal nodes, and lymphatic drainage continues inferiorly to the mediastinum. Running down the side of the thyroid gland is the recurrent laryngeal nerve.

ONCOLOGY

Thyroid cancer is rare, but it is the most common form of endocrine tumour. It is a disease that is slightly more common in women and can affect a wide range of ages, commonly between 25 and 65 years, with male cases tending to be older. The cause of thyroid cancer is unclear, but risk is greater in those individuals exposed to radiation. For example, more cases of thyroid cancer are seen in children who received radiotherapy at an early age and also after the Chernobyl nuclear disaster in the late 1980s and more recently the incident at the Fukushima nuclear reactor in Japan. Having a first-degree relative with thyroid cancer also increases the risk, and certain thyroid cancers are associated with a defective RET oncogene which can lead to multiple endocrine neoplasia (MEN) syndrome, which may run in families and can lead to medullary carcinoma.

Malignant tumours of the thyroid usually have one of four main histologies: papillary carcinoma, follicular carcinoma, medullary carcinoma or anaplastic carcinoma. Lymphomas and sarcomas are uncommon.

Papillary carcinoma is the most common form of thyroid cancer, most cases of which will present as multifocal disease throughout the thyroid gland. Spread to brain and bone does occur at a late stage, but more commonly spread is via the lymphatic system to the cervical lymph node chain.

Follicular carcinoma, along with papillary carcinoma, tends to be well differentiated, and about half of the tumours display the ability to utilise iodine to form thyroid hormone, although this occurs more commonly in follicular than in papillary tumours. Ingestion of radioiodine plays an important role in the treatment of patients with this condition. Normally, well-differentiated follicular tumours are well circumscribed. It is important at diagnosis to distinguish these from their benign counterpart, follicular adenoma. Spread to lymph nodes is fairly common, but this does not reduce survival. Follicular tumours readily spread via the blood to lungs and bone.

Medullary carcinoma arises from the parafollicular cells of the thyroid and constitutes 5% to 10% of all thyroid cancers. These cancers can be sporadic in nature and tend to be confined to one lobe of the thyroid. Medullary carcinoma may be familial in nature. These cancers are almost always bilateral at presentation and may be associated with MEN syndrome, in which other endocrine organs are affected. If familial medullary carcinoma is suspected, other members of the family should also be screened for disease. Familial medullary tumours may secrete calcitonin, which can be used as a tumour marker to monitor the efficacy of treatment. Spread to the cervical and mediastinal lymph nodes is common.

An anaplastic tumour is a highly aggressive, undifferentiated tumour. Spread via blood is early, but invasion of local tissues causes the main problems with this tumour. The trachea can be breached, causing stridor, or the oesophagus, causing dysphagia. Invasion of the recurrent laryngeal nerve may cause pain, and a breach of the carotid artery can cause death. Anaplastic tumours may be sub-classified into small cell and large cell. If small cell is suspected, this must be distinguished from lymphoma of the thyroid gland.

STAGING

The TNM staging system is often used, although this may be adapted depending on the histology of the disease. Importantly, the stage of the disease is based on the size of the tumour but also whether the tumour is confined to the thyroid or not. Any lymph node involvement will generally include the local paratracheal, pretrachael or prelaryngeal nodes, whilst more extensive nodal involvement might include the cervical lymph nodes.

Staging might also be adapted depending on the presenting histology and maybe even the age of the patient at presentation. Well-differentiated papillary and follicular thyroid cancer may be grouped according to whether the patient is under or over 55 years of age. Under 55 years only two stage groups are used, with stage I representing localised disease limited to the thyroid gland and stage II indicating wider disseminated disease. Over 55 years there are four stage groups more analogous to the traditional TNM system where stage I indicates localised, limited disease and stage IV indicates widespread metastases.

TREATMENT

Papillary and follicular tumours are best treated with surgery. Treatment may be lobectomy or total thyroidectomy and is largely dependent on the localised extent of the tumour along with the age of the patient and any co-morbidity. Because of the likely functioning nature of the disease, radioiodine may be administered to ablate any remaining thyroid tissue, in order to reduce the chance of recurrence. Lifelong supportive therapy in the form of replacement thyroid hormone is necessary.

Family members suspected of having medullary carcinoma should be screened for raised calcitonin level and the presence of the RET proto-oncogene as an important strategy for improved survival. Many patients with medullary carcinoma have lymph node spread to cervical and mediastinal regions. Total thyroidectomy is advocated for medullary carcinoma, along with en bloc neck dissection. These tumours are rarely functional; radioiodine has little efficacy.

Anaplastic tumours are locally very destructive. Surgery is advocated if the tumour remains localised, but this is rare. The most common treatment involves external beam radiotherapy.

Patients with well-differentiated tumours (normally papillary and follicular) have a favourable prognosis, with many surviving up to 10 years. Patients with anaplastic tumours have a poor survival rate. With medullary carcinoma, patients who have been diagnosed through screening have a better chance of survival.

Adrenal Glands

The adrenal glands are located immediately superior to the kidneys (Fig. 5.4). They are divided structurally and functionally into two parts: an outer section called the cortex and an inner one called the medulla.

The adrenal cortex secretes mainly glucocorticoid hormones such as hydrocortisone and cortisone. It also secretes aldosterone and small amounts of sex hormones. Over-secretion of these hormones is common in approximately 60% of adrenal cortex tumours, and patients may present with a variety of syndromes such as Cushing syndrome, adrenogenital syndrome, virilisation, hyperaldosteronism and feminisation. Adrenal cortex carcinoma is rare, with benign adenoma being far more common, and treatment consists mainly of surgery. Unfortunately, many malignant neoplasms will be locally invasive, with involvement of lymph nodes and direct extension to the renal vein being common occurrences. Postoperative radiotherapy has shown some benefit, as has the chemotherapy drug mitotane (Lysodren) for later stage disease.

The adrenal medulla secretes epinephrine (adrenaline) and norepinephrine (noradrenaline), which are hormones that act in the 'fight or flight' response of the body. Pheochromocytoma is the tumour most often identified in the adrenal medulla. Pheochromocytoma is often associated with increased secretion of the adrenal medulla hormones, and this is often used to diagnose the disease. Unfortunately, pheochromocytoma may be benign or malignant, and histologically it is difficult to tell them apart. Nevertheless, the treatment of choice is surgical removal, with associated regional lymph nodes if spread had been detected. Bilateral tumours affect a small percentage of patients, and these are usually associated with MEN, as outlined earlier. Identification of MEN calls for regular family screening for this disease.

STAGING

The stage of adrenal cortex tumours will influence any treatment given, which is usually surgery to remove the affected organ. TNM staging is based on the size – less than 5 cm for T1 or greater than 5 cm for T2 – but, importantly, any tumour must remain confined to the adrenal gland. Extension beyond the gland would constitute a later T stage and necessitate more involved surgery.

There is no TNM staging for tumours of the adrenal medulla at present.

PROGNOSIS

Patients diagnosed with adrenal gland tumours early have a good chance of survival. If spread is detected to local lymph nodes or further, the prognosis is worsened.

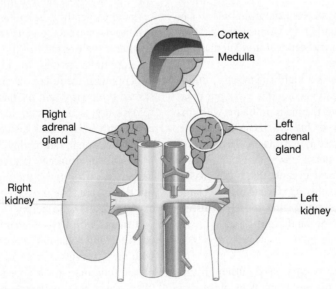

Fig. 5.4 The adrenal (suprarenal) glands.

SELF-ASSESSMENT QUESTIONS

Answer true or false to the following. Answers are on page 165–166.

1 *Endocrine glands secrete mucus.*

2 *The pituitary is situated below the optic chiasma.*

3 *The pituitary gland is situated in the sella turcica.*

4 *Virtually all tumours of the pituitary gland arise from the posterior lobe.*

5 *Most pituitary gland tumours are malignant.*

6 *Eosinophilic tumours often secrete growth hormone.*

7 *Surgery is the most common treatment for pituitary tumours.*

8 *The thyroid gland lies posterior to the larynx.*

9 *Lymphatic drainage of the thyroid is primarily to the cervical lymph node chain.*

10 *The thyroid gland uses thyroxine to produce its hormones.*

11 *Papillary carcinoma is the most common form of thyroid tumour.*

12 *Anaplastic tumours of the thyroid are usually very slow-growing.*

13 *Radioactive iodine is often used in the treatment of all thyroid tumours.*

14 *Medullary carcinoma of the thyroid has familial tendencies.*

15 *Papillary and follicular tumours of the thyroid are usually well differentiated.*

16 *Patients with well-differentiated tumours have a favourable prognosis.*

17 *The adrenal glands are located inferior to the kidneys.*

18 *The adrenal glands are divided into an outer cortex and an inner medulla.*

19 *Pheochromocytoma is a tumour most associated with the adrenal cortex.*

20 *Pheochromocytoma may be benign or malignant.*

Head and Neck Cancer

Chapter Outline

Objectives

By the end of this chapter, the reader should be able to:

- Describe the relational anatomy of the head and neck region.
- Understand the risk factors associated with head and neck cancer.
- Explain the signs and symptoms associated with the different types of pharyngeal cancers.
- Understand the role of epidermal growth factor receptor mutations in the development of and possible treatment for head and neck cancers.
- Describe the anatomy of the larynx and its relationship with staging for laryngeal cancer.
- Explain the role of surgery, chemotherapy, radiotherapy and biological therapies in the treatment of patients with head and neck cancer.

Head and neck cancer comprises malignancies within the head and neck region, and this chapter will cover cancers of the pharynx, oral cavity and larynx. These malignancies are often grouped together because of their anatomical site, histology and similar aetiology. Most patients with a suspected cancer within this region will be referred to a head and neck specialist.

Cancers of the head and neck tend to be squamous cell carcinoma (SCC) deriving from the stratified squamous epithelial that make up the mucosal lining of this area. Lymphoma (tonsils) and adenocarcinoma are rare. Importantly, 90% of head and neck squamous cell carcinomas (HNSCCS) will overexpress the epidermal growth factor receptor (EGFR), and this has led to the use of EGFR-directed therapies, such as cetuximab, in some cases, alongside radiotherapy. Aetiologically, risk of HNSCC is increased through excessive alcohol and tobacco consumption, and in the case of oral cavity and laryngeal cancers, the two combined will have a synergistic effect. Tobacco consumption will also include the use of smokeless tobacco products, such as snuff and chewing tobacco. Such risk factors may explain the increased risk in males. The chewing of areca nuts and betel quid, with or without tobacco, is a known risk factor and heightens the prevalence of oral cavity cancer in populations that partake of such habits. Oral cavity cancer is one of the most common cancers in India, where betel nut and areca nut consumption is commonplace.

Exposure to viral agents, such as the human papillomavirus (HPV) and Epstein–Barr virus (EBV), increases the risk of oropharyngeal and nasopharyngeal cancer, respectively. Persistent infection of HPV, mainly transmitted through oral sex, has led to an increase in HPV-positive HNSCC, and the oropharynx is the most common site for noncervical HPV-related cancer and in the absence of traditional risk factors, such as tobacco and alcohol use, represents the greatest risk. Interestingly, the median age of those with HPV-negative oropharyngeal cancer is around 65 years and is associated with the traditional risk factors, whereas in those with HPV-positive cancer, the median age is younger at around 53 years, representing a shift away from the traditional risk factors and heightened risk due to more sexual partners and earlier onset of sexual activity, thus increasing the risk of HPV infection. Furthermore, incidence is higher in among populations not vaccinated against HPV, suggesting that the HPV vaccination programme may reduce the risk for noncervical HPV-related cancers. Newly diagnosed patients with oropharyngeal cancers should be screened for HPV infection. Although this will not impact likely treatment options, it is known that HPV-positive patients have a better prognosis. Because post-treatment morbidity is a concern for patients with head and neck cancers, clinical trials are investigating whether less intensive treatments for HPV-positive cancer can deliver the same overall survival with less morbidity caused by intensive chemoradiation regimes.

Staging

The staging for head and neck cancers will be adapted for the various anatomical sites involved, and essentially the TNM is based around the size of the tumour within those sites. Some notable changes have occurred in the eighth edition TNM classification that have attempted to reflect changes in knowledge around these tumours. Firstly, the TNM now identifies HPV-positive oropharyngeal tumours as a separate pathology that, as such, demands its own codification. Secondly, extracapsular extension of lymph nodes for non-viral-associated HNSCC is seen as a detrimental prognostic indicator and, thirdly, the depth of invasion for oral cavity tumours should now be considered.

The Pharynx

Anatomically, the pharynx (Fig. 6.1) is divided into three sections. The nasopharynx lies posterior to the nasal cavity and extends from the base of the skull inferiorly to the level of the soft palate. It is continuous with the oropharynx, which lies posterior to the mouth and extends inferiorly to the level of the hyoid bone. Inferior to this is the laryngopharynx (hypopharynx), which extends from the level of the hyoid bone to its termination in the oesophagus, posterior to the larynx.

Several openings can be found in the pharynx:
- right and left auditory tubes opening into the nasopharynx
- two posterior nares from the nasal cavity into the nasopharynx
- the opening of the mouth (fauces) into the oropharynx
- the opening of the larynx and oesophagus from the laryngopharynx.

Each of these openings plays a part in the potential spread of tumours within this region, and the signs and symptoms with which patients present can often be traced back to involvement of these structures. Similarly, there is a deep depression posterior to the openings of the auditory tubes called the fossa of Rosenmüller, and this is a common site of presentation of nasopharyngeal tumours.

Functionally, the pharynx plays a role in both the respiratory and digestive systems. It also plays an important part in the creation of sounds.

An important source of aggregated lymphatic tissue, collectively known as the tonsils, is located in this region. Three pairs of tonsils, sometimes referred to as Waldeyer ring, protect the passageway from harmful micro-organisms. The pharyngeal tonsils are located on the posterior wall of the nasopharynx opposite the posterior nares. The palatine tonsils in the oropharynx are located behind and below the pillars of fauces,

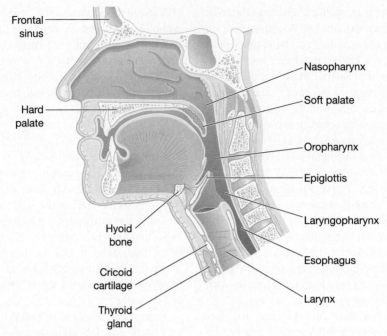

Fig. 6.1 The relational anatomy of the pharynx.

and the lingual tonsils are located at the base of the tongue. The epithelial lining of the pharynx changes slightly from a pseudostratified ciliated columnar form in the nasopharynx to a stratified squamous form in the laryngopharynx.

The pharynx has a rich lymphatic drainage and, as a result, early lymphatic involvement is common. Of importance is the node of Rouviere, which is found in the lateral aspect of the retropharyngeal wall and is a point of early involvement, particularly for nasopharyngeal tumours. Other directions of lymphatic spread can be to the jugulodigastric nodes, jugulo-omohyoid, deep cervical chain, and posterior triangle.

Oncology

NASOPHARYNGEAL CARCINOMA

Nasopharyngeal carcinoma is rare in most parts of the world but is relatively common in parts of Southeast Asia. The highest incidence worldwide occurs in Asia and North Africa, with salted fish containing nitrates being the main causative factor. Many cancers of the

nasopharynx will be associated with EBV infection, and in rare cases, nasopharyngeal carcinoma may run in families. Possible causes include exposure to nitrosamines, polycyclic hydrocarbons, chronic nasal infection, poor hygiene and poor ventilation of the nasopharynx, and smoking will also increase risk. Generally, more males than females are affected.

The main presenting pathology is SCC, although this cell type is often subdivided into well-differentiated (keratinising) and poorly differentiated (nonkeratinising) tumours, with anaplastic tumours making up a third variety. Tumours that have lymphocyte involvement may be referred to as lymphoepithelioma. Because there is also an abundance of lymphatic tissue in this region, lymphomas, usually of the non-Hodgkin variety, are also quite common.

Patients may present with a variety of signs and symptoms. Occlusion of the eustachian tube may lead to hearing difficulties, cranial nerve dysfunction (usually II–VI or IX–XII), enlarged cervical lymph nodes (which may be bilateral because of the cross-lymphatic drainage of this area), sore throat, epistaxis or blocked nose.

Staging

Staging for nasopharyngeal tumours is based on the level of extension within, or beyond, the nasopharynx, with early stage representing disease contained within this region and later stage representing extension beyond and maybe into the bone of the skull. Lymph node involvement is common, and laterality as well as the size (smaller or greater than 6 cm in diameter) of the involved lymph node(s) is important.

Treatment

Radiotherapy remains the treatment of choice for tumours in the nasopharyngeal region, whether of squamous epithelial type or lymphomas. Generally, SCCs will receive higher doses of radiation than lymphomas. Radiotherapy for SCCs tends to involve the primary site along with potential routes of spread. The upper deep cervical lymph node chain should be included in the field along with the nodes of the posterior triangle and lateral pharyngeal area. Both sides of the head and neck should be treated because of the likelihood of cross-lymphatic spread.

Often, for stage 3 (sometimes 2) and above, chemotherapy alongside the radiotherapy, termed chemoradiation, will be used. Generally, platinum-based drugs, such as cisplatin or carboplatin, are the drugs used due to their radio-sensitising nature.

Sometimes brachytherapy is used to boost the dose to the primary site. The relatively inaccessible nature of the nasopharynx makes this a difficult procedure, and treatment of this type should only be attempted in specialised centres. Any surgical procedures are normally limited to biopsy and maybe removal of affected lymph nodes.

Prognosis

Patients with early-stage disease survive longer with 5-year survival rates around 85% for localised disease, and this will fall to around 70% for locoregional involvement and 50% for distant disease.

OROPHARYNGEAL CARCINOMA

Oropharyngeal carcinoma is also a rare disease in the UK. It is predominantly a disease of the elderly (median age is about 65 years). It is far more common in males than in females, which may be related to habitual smoking and high alcohol intake. SCC is the predominant pathology. However, because of the abundance of lymphoid tissue present, non-Hodgkin lymphomas are also quite common.

Patients may present with a variety of symptoms mainly associated with the tumour site of presentation and local spread of the tumour. Base of tongue tumours may produce fixation of the tongue, resulting in slurring of speech. Referred pain to the ears may occur if spread superior to the eustachian tubes is present. Tonsillar tumours tend to present with no or mild pain and dysphagia as the tumour begins to occlude the passageway. Early lymph spread is common, with many patients presenting with node enlargement in the neck, some of which may be bilateral.

Staging

TNM definitions and stage groups for oropharyngeal carcinoma are different for HPV-positive and HPV-negative disease. Generally, the T classification remains identical and is based primarily on size. Extension and deeper invasion into surrounding structures would indicate a higher T classification. The interesting difference in the staging lies within the lymph node classification. Clinical lymph node status takes into account, size, laterality and extranodal extension. Table 6.1 outlines the important differences.

TABLE 6.1 **Lymph Node Staging for Oropharyngeal Tumours by HPV Status**		
	HPV−ve	**HPV+ve**
N1	Ipsilateral, single <3 cm	Unilateral ≤6 cm
N2	Single or multiple, ipsilateral <3 cm, >6 cm. Bilateral or contralateral may indicate N2c.	Contralateral or bilateral ≤6 cm
N3	(a) >6 cm (b) Single or multiple with extranodal involvement	>6 cm
pN	Pathological assessment of size and any extranodal involvement	Pathological assessment will determine the number of lymph nodes involved.

HPV, Human papillomavirus.

It is important to note here that HPV+ve tumours tend to have a more favourable prognosis and therefore larger lymph node involvement will not necessarily impact on outcome. Also of interest is the wording. HPV−ve indicates that for N1 status, the affected lymph nodes should be on the same side as the presenting tumour (ipsilateral), whereas HPV+ve indicates "unilateral," meaning affected lymph nodes are all on "one side," but not necessarily the same side. Laterality is difficult to assess sometimes, particularly if a midline structure is involved, but is important to assess as accurately as possible because of its impact on likely treatment, in particular radiotherapy, which will be used to treat any lymph node involvement. Radiotherapy to only the affected side may lead to a decrease in radiation-induced side effects and a better quality of life for those affected.

Treatment

Treatment will generally involve a combination of surgery, radiotherapy and maybe chemotherapy. Surgery is the initial treatment and may be the only treatment required for early-stage tumours. Generally, radiotherapy will be used adjuvantly, particularly if the tumour could not be fully removed and lymph node involvement is suspected. Often, for locally advanced tumours, chemotherapy will be used alongside the radiotherapy, and cisplatin with or without 5FU is the drug used. For those tumours that demonstrate EGFR positivity, the monoclonal antibody cetuximab may be used, either alongside radiotherapy or in combination with chemotherapy for advanced stages.

Prognosis

Those with early-stage tumours will have better survival, with around 80% surviving more than 3 years. This falls to around 50% for later stages. Morbidity associated with the aggressive treatments is a source for debate at present, with many survivors experiencing the often devastating effects of treatments such as surgery and radiotherapy. Both physical and psychological trauma have given rise to higher-than-normal suicide rates in survivors of head and neck cancers. Research is being undertaken to see if less intensive treatments can be given to those with a better prognosis whilst still achieving the same or better outcomes in terms of survival; for example, those with HPV+ve oropharyngeal cancers. Patients who continue to smoke during or after radiotherapy tend to have a worse outcome with greater chance of recurrence.

LARYNGOPHARYNGEAL (HYPOPHARYNGEAL) CARCINOMA

The laryngopharynx, or hypopharynx, extends from the plane of the hyoid bone distally to the plane of the lower border of the cricoid cartilage. It does not include the larynx per se but does include the posterior aspect that is continuous with the oesophagus. As a consequence, invasion into the larynx may occur, and this will inform staging criteria. The hypopharynx has three parts: the pyriform fossa, the postcricoid area and the posterior pharyngeal wall. The pyriform fossa is the most frequently involved site in the laryngopharynx. Postcricoid and posterior laryngopharyngeal wall carcinomas account for only one-third of laryngopharyngeal cancers.

When involved by cancer, this anatomical region does not generate symptoms until late in the course of the disease. In addition to having a high incidence of early metastases, tumours of the laryngopharynx have survival rates that are perhaps the lowest of all sites in the head and neck. The predominant cell type is SCC, often with multiple sites being involved. Presentation is associated with a history of excess use of tobacco or alcohol, and co-morbidity often associated with these, such as lung and liver disease, will have a bearing on any possible treatment strategy and likely outcome.

Lymph node involvement is frequent, particularly the cervical lymph node chain, and examination of the regional lymph nodes (jugulodigastric, juguloomohyoid, upper and middle deep cervical and retropharyngeal nodes) pathologically is essential for accurate staging.

Staging

The T classification for these tumours is primarily based on the size of the tumour and involvement of one or more of the subsites above. Invasion into and fixation of the hemilarynx, oesophagus or other structures, such as the hyoid bone or thyroid cartilage, points to late-stage disease. Lymph node involvement is common and both clinical and pathological assessment is done as for oropharyngeal (HPV−ve) tumours above.

Treatment

Because of the nature of this disease and its lack of symptoms until late in its course, it is unusual to have patients with early-stage disease. As a consequence, the tumour tends to invade locally and early via the lymphatic system. Surgery is the mainstay of treatment for these patients, with total laryngopharyngectomy and neck dissection being the norm. For later stage disease, postoperative radiotherapy may be used. Neo-adjuvant chemotherapy is sometimes used to shrink the tumour prior to administering other forms of treatment, with cisplatin in combination with 5FU being the most likely used drug. Radiotherapy is generally less effective for patients who continue to smoke during treatment and, as such, these patients tend to have lower response rates and poorer survival.

Oral Cavity

The oral cavity extends from the vermilion border of the lip (where the skin of the face meets the true lip) to the junction of the hard and soft palate superiorly and to the line of circumvallate papillae (taste buds) inferiorly. The oral cavity is divided into the lips, tongue, buccal (cheek) mucosa, floor of the mouth, gingiva (gums) and hard palate. The three sets of tonsils, palatine, pharyngeal and lingua, are found at the back of the oral cavity where it extends into the oropharynx (Fig. 6.2).

Many structures within the head and neck share lymphatic drainage, and an understanding of where tumours are likely to spread is of vital importance in the management of head and neck tumours. The main routes of lymphatic drainage for this anatomic area are to the buccinator, jugulodigastric, submandibular and submental nodes initially (Fig. 6.3). Subsequent lymphatic drainage includes the parotid and jugular nodes, as well as the upper and lower cervical chain of nodes.

ONCOLOGY

The oral cavity is lined with a mucous membrane composed of squamous epithelium; consequently, the majority of tumours in this area are SCCs. Tobacco smoking and drinking alcohol are the two main risk factors associated with oral cavity cancer. Smoking and drinking to excess have a synergistic effect where the overall risk is greater than the sum of the individual risks associated with smoking and drinking. Oral tobacco products, such as chewing tobacco, snuff and betel quid, are also associated with increased risk. Overexposure to sunlight (UV radiation) is implicated in lip cancer. Certain conditions, such as leukoplakia, characterised by a white furry patch, or erythroplakia, a red-coloured patch, on the inside of the mouth are thought to be pre-cancerous conditions and will often be removed by surgery.

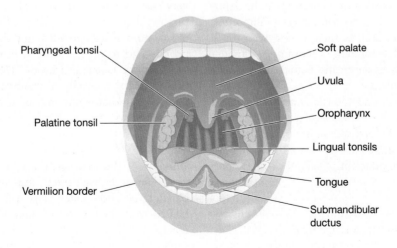

Fig. 6.2 The oral cavity.

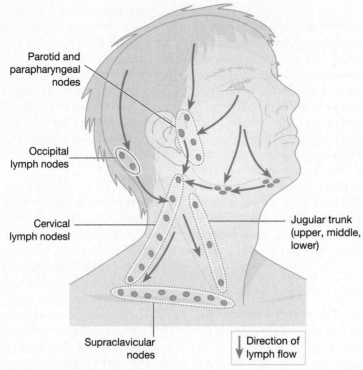

Fig. 6.3 Lymph node drainage of the head and neck.

Staging

The TNM staging for oral cavity tumours is primarily based on the size of the tumour, and accurate assessment of lymph node involvement is essential and will affect treatment and probably outcome. Recent revision of the TNM classification indicates that the depth of involvement of oral cavity tumours is an important prognostic indicator and, as such, is now with the T classification for these tumours. For example, tumours with a depth of invasion greater than 10 mm would indicate T3 or T4 disease.

Lymph node assessment is vital, and both sides of the head and neck should be investigated, as laterality will influence the N classification. Important here also is whether or not extranodal involvement is present, with presence often indicating a later N classification.

The Lip

Lip cancers comprise approximately 25% of oral cavity tumours and are predominantly SCCs. Males are much more likely to get lip cancer, probably because

of smoking. Exposure to sunlight is also implicated and a reason why the lower lip is often more affected than the upper lip, which generally is afforded more protection.

Interestingly, basal cell carcinoma of the lip is very rare. Where the lip is involved with this type of tumour, it is more often than not the case that a skin of face tumour has extended onto the lip. Fortunately, people tend to present early with cancer of the lip, probably for cosmetic reasons. This early presentation means that results of treatment are very good. Surgery or radiotherapy may be used either alone or in combination.

The Oral Cavity

Tumours of the oral cavity are generally SCCs and treated using either surgery, radiotherapy or a combination of both. Later stage cancer may also be treated with chemotherapy alongside EGFR-directed therapies such as cetuximab or immunotherapy drugs such as nivolumab. One of the significant factors in choosing treatment is the anticipated functional deficit that surgery may involve.

Early stage tumours tend to be surgically removed. Patients with later stage disease will often have a combination of surgery and radiotherapy. It is most important that possible routes of lymphatic spread be fully examined and, if positive, included in any treatment of the patient. This may involve block dissection of the nodes or inclusion of the lymphatic drainage in the radiotherapy treatment field.

Survival is better for those with early-stage disease, with 5-year survival dropping to around 50% for those with late-stage disease. As discussed earlier, treatment-associated morbidity is an area of much debate, and survivors need as good a quality of life as possible.

The Tongue

The tongue is a solid mass of skeletal muscle that is covered with a mucous membrane. Its muscles run in many directions, giving it the high manoeuvrability that is required in the processes of both mastication and phonation. It has a blunt root that inserts into the back of the oral cavity, a tip and a central body. Descriptively and oncologically, the tongue can be divided into the anterior two-thirds and the posterior third, separated by the sulcus terminalis, a V-shaped line on the dorsal aspect (Fig. 6.4). The surface of anterior two-thirds' is moist and covered with papillae (taste buds).

Approximately 75% of all tongue tumours, the majority of which are SCCs, with the occasional adenocarcinoma, arise on the anterior two-thirds. Extension of the tongue outside the oral cavity means that there is good accessibility for surgical techniques. These tumours may be treated with radiotherapy, surgery-or a combination. The aim of any treatment is to offer a good chance of cure while maintaining function, wherever possible.

Posterior third tumours of the tongue warrant a different management approach. This part of the tongue comprises lymphatic tissue called the lingual tonsils. The common histology is lymphoma, most commonly non-Hodgkin lymphoma (see Chapter 2). Because these tumours are highly radiosensitive, they often receive external beam radiotherapy, which uses large fields to include the primary site and associated lymphatic drainage.

It is important to note that patients who continue to smoke while receiving radiation therapy for oral cavity tumours appear to have lower response rates and shorter survival times than those who do not.

The Larynx

The larynx or voice box (Fig. 6.5) lies below the hyoid bone, anterior to the oesophagus and continuous with the trachea. It is supported by cartilage and contains the vocal fold (vocal cords). The function of the larynx is to produce sound that varies in pitch. This is achieved by varying the tension of the ligaments within the vocal fold. The width of the slit between the vocal folds can also be varied by movement of the arytenoid cartilages brought about by the vocal muscles.

Anatomically, the larynx is divided into three regions. The supraglottic region (supraglottis) includes the epiglottis, false vocal cords, ventricles, aryepiglottic folds and arytenoids. The glottic region (glottis) includes the true vocal cords and the anterior and posterior commissures. The subglottic region (subglottis) begins about 1 cm below the true vocal cords and extends to the lower border of the cricoid cartilage.

Knowledge of the lymphatic drainage of the larynx is important in understanding the presentation and associated management of malignant disease arising in this area. The true vocal cords have sparse lymphatic drainage, which explains why true vocal cord tumours rarely present with cervical lymph node enlargement. By contrast, the supraglottic and subglottic regions have a rich lymphatic network. The supraglottic region drains principally to the upper deep cervical lymph node chain, and a great proportion of patients with malignant disease will present with enlarged nodes. The subglottic region drains to the paratracheal and lower cervical nodes.

ONCOLOGY

Cancer of the larynx is one of the most common head and neck cancers in Europe. Because changes in voice and a sore throat tend to be common presenting symptoms, patients are likely to seek medical advice early, meaning most patients tend to present with early-stage disease. Approximately three-quarters of tumours will occur in the glottic region (vocal folds) of the larynx. Laryngeal cancer affects more men than women, and important causative factors are smoking and excessive alcohol intake. Patients who continue to smoke

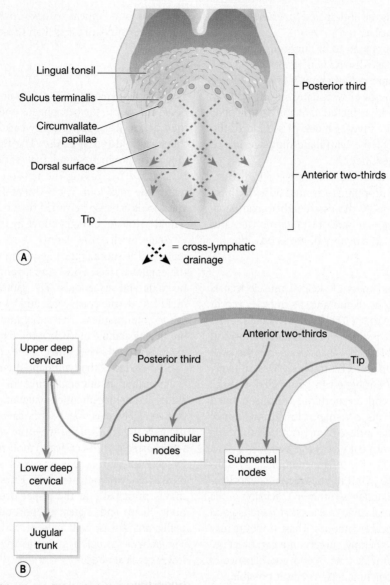

Fig. 6.4 (A) Anatomy of the tongue. (B) Lymphatic drainage of the tongue.

and drink alcohol during treatment tend to have a decreased chance of cure and an increased risk of a second cancer. HPV has also been implicated in some tumours.

Pathologically, the principal histology is SCC; these may be keratinising or nonkeratinising, well or poorly differentiated. The majority of glottic tumours arise in the anterior portion of the vocal cord, with frequent involvement of the anterior commissure.

Staging

It is important to obtain the most accurate clinical staging for these tumours, as this will ultimately affect the management of the patient. Clinical examination, followed by direct or indirect laryngoscopy, is essential. Biopsy will provide information about the grade of the tumour, and computed tomography (CT) or magnetic resonance imaging (MRI) will also help diagnose the extent of tumour spread.

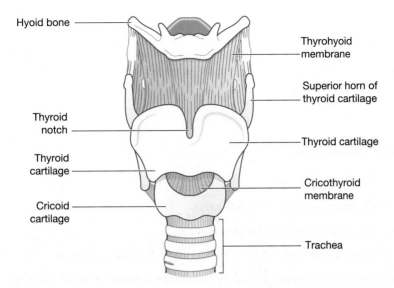

Hyoid bone

Thyrohyoid membrane

Superior horn of thyroid cartilage

Thyroid notch

Thyroid cartilage

Thyroid cartilage

Cricothyroid membrane

Cricoid cartilage

Trachea

Fig. 6.5 Anatomy of the larynx.

TNM staging for these cancers will be influenced by region involved (glottis, sub- or supraglottis), whether one or both cords are affected, whether those cords are fixed or mobile and lymph node involvement (laterality and whether there is evidence of extra-nodal extension).

Treatment

Superficial tumours confined to the larynx without fixation or lymphatic spread can be cured by either radiotherapy or surgery. Because true glottic tumours have very little chance of spreading lymphatically, there is no need to include the cervical lymph node chain in a radiotherapy treatment field, which usually includes the whole of the larynx. Small tumours confined to the cord may also be treated successfully with a variety of surgical techniques, such as cordectomy and laser microsurgery. The overriding factor in choice of treatment is likelihood of success while maintaining the function of the larynx. Larger, T2 or supraglottic tumours can also be treated successfully with radiotherapy. It is important to electively treat the cervical lymph node chain on both sides of the neck. For patients with cancer of the subglottis, combined modality therapy is generally preferred, although for the uncommon small lesions (stage I or stage II), radiation therapy alone may be used. Patients who continue to smoke throughout their treatment have significantly less chance of success and therefore should be encouraged to stop smoking. For later stage disease, radiotherapy may be the preferred option of treatment, with surgery available as a back-up if radiotherapy is unsuccessful.

Prognosis

Prognosis is very much influenced by the T and N stage of the disease. Small tumours with no lymph node involvement have a very high chance of cure. Locally advanced lesions with large lymph nodes respond poorly to any form of treatment and consequently have a poor prognosis. Patients treated for laryngeal cancers are at highest risk of recurrence in the first 2 to 3 years. Recurrences after 5 years are rare.

General Note on Head and Neck Cancer

Treatment for head and neck cancer offers many challenges from both functional and cosmetic points of view. Importantly, much attention has now fallen on survivorship and living beyond cancer. Surgery for these cancers can often involve extremely invasive procedures that can lead to disfigurement and dysfunction. Alongside this, high-dose radiotherapy to the head and neck region can cause severe radiation reactions that can persist for many years.

The idea behind treatment is to always offer success whilst maintaining function; however, many patients living beyond treatment often face years of complications brought on by the treatments. Loneliness and a feeling of helplessness are often reported by these patients, and unfortunately, suicide rates amongst this group of survivors are higher than average. Research needs to persist in order to achieve optimum results whilst also maintaining the quality of life for these patients and realisation that extra support and care is needed long after treatment has finished.

SELF-ASSESSMENT QUESTIONS

Answer true or false to the following. Answers are on page 165–166.

1 *Most head and neck cancers will be adenocarcinomas.*

2 *EGFR is often overexpressed in head and neck cancers.*

3 *The nasopharynx extends from the base of the skull to the level of the hyoid bone.*

4 *The fossa of Rosenmüller is a common place for presentation of nasopharyngeal tumours.*

5 *Staging for nasopharyngeal tumours is based on the level of extension within or beyond the nasopharynx.*

6 *Surgery is the most common treatment for nasopharyngeal tumours.*

7 *The oropharynx contains three pairs of tonsils.*

8 *Persistent HPV infection can increase the risk of oropharyngeal cancer.*

9 *HPV+ve and HPV−ve tumours are staged identically.*

10 *Cetuximab is often used in combination with chemotherapy to treat late-stage head and neck cancers.*

11 *Patients with HPV+ve oropharyngeal cancers have a better prognosis than those with HPV−ve cancers.*

12 *Patients with laryngopharyngeal cancer generally have a good prognosis.*

13 *Pyriform fossa tumours make up the majority of laryngopharynx tumours.*

14 *Excessive alcohol intake and tobacco consumption are the main risk factors for oral cavity cancers.*

15 *Lymph from the anterior two-thirds of the tongue goes straight to the cervical lymph nodes.*

16 *Most tongue cancers are SCCs.*

17 *The larynx is divided into three regions: the supraglottic, glottic and subglottic.*

18 *Glottic tumours tend to present early with cervical lymph node enlargement.*

19 *Patients who drink and smoke while undergoing treatment for a larynx tumour have a decreased chance of cure.*

20 *T1 glottic tumours suggest that the vocal cords are immobile.*

Digestive System Tumours

Chapter Outline

Objectives

By the end of this chapter, the reader should be able to:

- Identify the key organs of the gastrointestinal tract and outline their functions.
- Outline the risk factors associated with cancers of the gastrointestinal tract.
- Outline the principles of TNM staging for cancers of the gastrointestinal tract.
- Describe the principles underpinning screening for bowel cancer.
- Understand the role of EGFR, KRAS, HER2 and other genetic mutations found in cancers of the gastrointestinal tract and how they relate to possible treatment options.
- Outline the role of surgery, chemotherapy, radiotherapy and biological therapies in the treatment of patients for gastrointestinal tract tumours.

The digestive system is concerned with the ingestion, digestion and absorption of nutrients that can be used for metabolic processes by living cells. It is composed of numerous organs (Fig. 7.1). Some, such as the stomach and intestine, have a direct effect on the absorption of foodstuffs. Others, such as the pancreas, liver and gallbladder, have an indirect effect and are termed accessory organs because they produce secretions that are transported to the intestines to aid the breakdown of food. For oral cavity tumours, see Chapter 6.

Oesophagus

The oesophagus is a tube that extends from the pharynx to the stomach, allowing the passage of food. It is approximately 25 cm long and lies immediately posterior to the trachealis muscle of the trachea

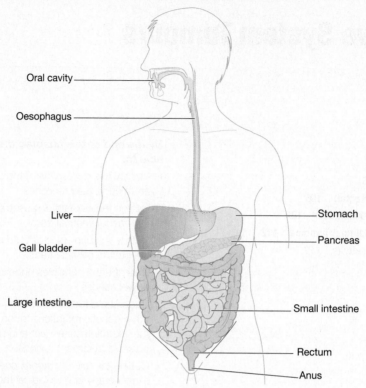

Fig. 7.1 Organs of the digestive system.

(a possible route of tumour spread) and anterior to the cervical and thoracic vertebrae. Flat when not in use, it is able to distend into the space occupied by the soft trachealis muscle, to accommodate a bolus of food. The oesophagus has an abrasion-resistant lining surrounded by layers of striated muscle. The oesophagus can conveniently be divided into three sections: upper, middle and lower. The mucosa is made up mainly of stratified squamous epithelium. Changes (metaplasia) may happen because of acid reflux that results in more glandular-like epithelium, especially in the lower third. Such changes can give rise to a condition known as Barrett oesophagus, a known precursor to oesophageal cancer. The oesophagus enters the stomach at the cardia through the cardiac sphincter.

ONCOLOGY

Oesophageal cancer is more common in males and usually occurs in the 60 to 80 years of age group. It is rare below 50 years of age and tends to affect those in lower socioeconomic groups. The incidence

of oesophageal cancer continues to rise and whereas previously most cancers were SCCs arising from the stratified squamous epithelium of the upper and middle thirds of the oesophagus, this distribution is beginning to change. Adenocarcinomas arising mainly at the lower third region are now the predominant histology, particularly in the United States and Western Europe. Smoking and drinking (the two together exhibit synergism) have been widely associated with increased risk of oesophageal cancer, especially squamous cell carcinoma. Poor diet and male obesity are also known risk factors for adenocarcinoma of the oesophagus, mainly because of the increased risk of acid reflux. The rise in incidence of Barrett oesophagus may also offer a useful explanation as to the increase in incidence for lower third adenocarcinomas. Long-term regurgitation of stomach contents into the lower third of the oesophagus may lead to dysplastic changes that result in Barrett oesophagus, which is thought to be a risk factor in developing adenocarcinoma of the lower oesophagus.

Staging

Staging of oesophageal tumours is primarily based on the level of infiltration through the muscle layer of the oesophagus. An oesophageal tumour is likely to spread microscopically along and around the lumen of the oesophagus (Fig. 7.2), leading to the patient presenting with progressive dysphagia, usually resulting in massive weight loss. Patients tend to be very undernourished and dehydrated. The location of the tumour will influence the likely lymphatic spread of the tumour, with upper third tumours draining to the paratracheal and supraclavicular nodes, middle third tumours draining to the hilar and mediastinal nodes and lower third tumours draining to the paraesophageal and gastric nodes. Because the oesophagus is the first part of the digestive tube proper, its blood will ultimately go to the liver, a likely route of spread.

Treatment

Treatment of oesophageal cancer is based on whether a cure or palliation is intended. For very early-stage lesions, which are rare, endoscopic mucosal resection may be an option. Surgery is curative for those patients with localised disease, the extent of which, partial or total oesophagectomy, will be determined by patient choice and perceived post-surgical quality of life. Radiotherapy may be an option for patients unfit for surgery but only for localised disease. For patients with advanced disease, a combination of surgery and chemotherapy is the treatment of choice. Chemotherapy usually involves a combination of platinum-based drugs, such as cisplatin and 5 fluorouracil (5FU), which may be given neo-adjuvantly in some cases. Palliation through stenting may also be considered. Unfortunately, results of treatment are poor for this type of cancer, with few patients surviving 5 years.

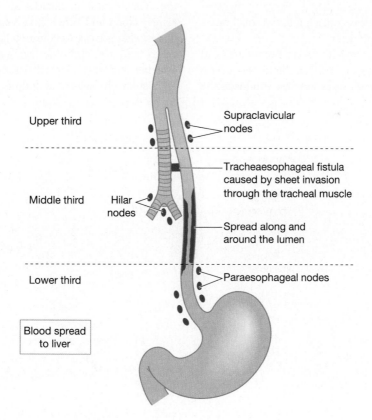

Upper third

Supraclavicular nodes

Tracheaesophageal fistula caused by sheet invasion through the tracheal muscle

Middle third

Hilar nodes

Spread along and around the lumen

Lower third

Paraesophageal nodes

Blood spread to liver

Fig. 7.2 Possible routes of spread for oesophageal tumours.

Stomach

The stomach lies mainly in the left upper quadrant of the abdomen between the oesophagus and small intestine. It is normally J-shaped and has a greater curvature and a lesser curvature (Fig. 7.3). The right part of the stomach lies under the liver; the left part is under the diaphragm, upon which the left lung sits. The stomach acts mainly as a storage area and can distend to accommodate large quantities of food. This distension occurs mainly at the superior portion of the stomach and therefore restricts the potential movement of the lungs inferiorly, giving the feeling of shortness of breath after overeating. Anatomically, the stomach is divided into various sections. The cardiac region, where the oesophagus enters, is bordered by the cardiac sphincter (valve), which allows foodstuffs to pass into the stomach but not back into the oesophagus. Heartburn is caused by reflux of the acidic contents of the stomach back through this sphincter and burning of the lower oesophagus. Partially digested foodstuff passes from the stomach into the small intestine via the pyloric sphincter.

The fundus of the stomach acts as a storage area and is the part that pushes upwards on the under-surface of the diaphragm. Food moves from the fundus to the body of the stomach, a central portion where food is churned and mixed with the gastric secretions. The final section is the pylorus, the distal end of the stomach that joins the duodenum via the pyloric sphincter. The mucosa of the stomach is lined with simple columnar epithelium containing large numbers of gastric glands. These glands secrete most of the gastric juice, a mucus-type fluid containing enzymes and hydrochloric acid. The stomach is a highly muscular organ with longitudinal, circular and oblique muscle fibres allowing the stomach to contract in different directions so that the food is broken up and mixed effectively. The lining of the stomach and remainder of the digestive system contain aggregated lymphatic tissue, and local lymphatic drainage is to the gastric and splenic nodes.

ONCOLOGY

Worldwide, cancer of the stomach is still a significant health risk, although generally the incidence is declining. The highest incidences are recorded in South Korea, Japan and other East Asian countries. It is a disease that is twice as common in men, although this varies with age, and older age groups generally have a higher incidence. Several risk factors are associated with stomach cancer, including *Helicobacter pylori*

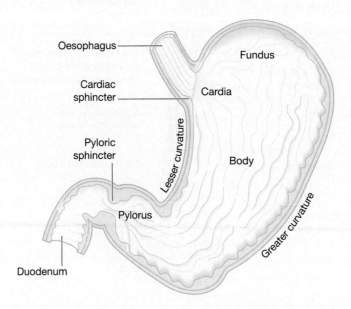

Fig. 7.3 The stomach.

infection, a diet including dry salted foods, atrophic gastritis, pernicious anaemia and cigarette smoking, and 1% to 3% of cases may be hereditary. Multiple daily rations of fruit and vegetables may have a preventive effect, along with vitamin C.

Most tumours of the stomach are adenocarcinomas and may be subdivided into intestinal (well-differentiated) and diffuse (poorly differentiated) tumours, with the latter tending to be more invasive with a higher propensity to spread. With carcinoid tumours (see later), lymphomas and leiomyosarcomas making up the rest of the histologies, tumours may also be assessed for both HER2 and PD1/PDL1 overexpression.

Endoscopic examination with biopsy will be the main investigative technique. A staging endoscopic ultrasound may be used, along with CT and maybe PET scans, to ascertain the level of invasion of any lesion. Staging is determined by the extent of invasion into the muscle layer of the stomach. Spread is to the regional lymphatics, which do have a bearing on the prognosis for the patient. Blood spread is possible and usually involves the liver. Invasion through the stomach wall may lead to peritoneal metastases. Unfortunately, because of the ability of the stomach to distend with minimal discomfort, and that over 50% of patients will present with late stage disease, overall prognosis is poor.

Staging

The TNM staging for stomach cancer is based around the level of invasion of the tumour. Early stage will have disease limited to the mucosa, with stage IV demonstrating that the tumour has invaded all the way through the wall of the stomach, maybe even involving other structures in the immediate vicinity.

Treatment

Due to the late presentation, very few patients are eligible for radical surgery, which represents the best chance of cure. However, partial gastrectomy and laser therapy play an important role in palliation of symptoms. Because of the radiosensitive nature of the stomach mucosa, radiotherapy can only be tolerated in small doses, and it therefore tends to be reserved for palliative rather than curative treatment. Chemotherapy (epirubicin, cisplatin, 5FU),

alone or in combination with radiotherapy or surgery, may be used in late-stage disease. Those with late-stage disease with overexpressed HER2 may also be given trastuzumab (Herceptin), and those with PD1/PDL1 overexpression may be offered immunotherapy checkpoint inhibitor drugs, such as nivolumab.

Survival is very much based on stage. Around 35% to 65% of patients with earlier stage disease will survive 5 years, and this falls to less than 25% for stage III, and unfortunately, very few with stage IV will survive longer than a year.

Small Intestine

The small intestine (or small bowel) is approximately 6.5 m long and consists of the duodenum (25 cm), jejunum (2.5 m) and ileum (3.6 m). Its coiled loops fill most of the abdominal cavity. The duodenum is the uppermost section and a continuation from the pylorus of the stomach. It is shaped like a letter C, surrounds the head of the pancreas and receives the common bile duct (from the gallbladder and liver) and the pancreatic duct at a small, raised area called the hepatopancreatic ampulla (ampulla of Vater). The mucosal layer is epithelial and lined with many glands that secrete intestinal juice, although some cells are specialised and secrete mucus (goblet cells). Other cells called enteroendocrine cells have a more endocrine function and produce hormones that stimulate the secretion of bicarbonated pancreatic juice to balance the intestinal pH against the effect of acidic chyme from the stomach. Enterochromaffin cells, a particular type of enteroendocrine cell, secrete serotonin and may develop into a particular type of cancer called a carcinoid tumour (see later) within the small intestine. Scattered throughout the mucous membrane are solitary lymphatic nodules, most numerous in the lower part of the ileum. These may be joined together to form aggregated lymphatic nodules (Peyer patches) that protect the intestines from ingested microbes and dirt. The main purpose of the small intestine is to absorb the nutrients from food. Thus, it has a rich blood supply, and all blood from this part of the body is transported directly to the liver as part of the hepatic circulation, so liver metastasis is a common form of spread for intestinal cancer.

ONCOLOGY

Cancer of the small intestine accounts for only a small percentage of gastrointestinal malignancies (1% to 2%). Different histologies tend to be present in the various parts of the small intestine, with adenocarcinoma being the main tumour type associated with the duodenum and first part of the jejunum. Lymphomas are rare in this section but relatively common in the ileum, along with carcinoid tumours. Rarely, leiomyosarcomas can also be found in the small intestine. Patients may present with a variety of symptoms, mainly due to obstruction, with a sense of abdominal discomfort. The length of the small intestine, along with the rich blood supply, often means that patients present with late-stage disease, with stage being based on the level of invasion through the wall of the intestine. Curability is directly associated with the resectability of the tumour and its histology. Patients with leiomyosarcoma generally fare better than those with adenocarcinoma. Surgery is the main form of curative treatment available, maybe in combination with chemotherapy.

Large Intestine (Colorectal)

The large intestine (or large bowel – Fig. 7.4) is about 1.5 m long. It is continuous with the ileum, where it becomes the caecum. The caecum is continuous upwards with the ascending colon, which turns sharply towards midline at the hepatic flexure to become the transverse colon. This, in turn, is deflected downwards by the spleen at the splenic flexure. This downward segment is called the descending colon. Onwards, the colon forms an S-shaped curve known as the sigmoid colon before terminating at the rectum and anus. The large intestine is lined with columnar epithelium and mucus-secreting goblet cells. Its primary function is to absorb water.

ONCOLOGY

Cancer of the large intestine, termed colorectal cancer, affects a significant number of people in developed countries. It is the second most common cancer in the United States and fourth in the United Kingdom and is generally more common in males. Adenocarcinomas are the most common type, constituting approximately 90% of cases, with carcinoid tumours and leiomyosarcomas making up the rest. The greatest proportion of cases occur in the sigmoid colon, followed closely by the rectum and caecum areas. A large proportion of colorectal cancers may be associated with poor diet incorporating increased amounts of red and processed meats, increased alcohol consumption, physical inactivity resulting in reduced peristaltic activity, obesity and smoking. Such risk factors explain why colorectal cancer tends to be

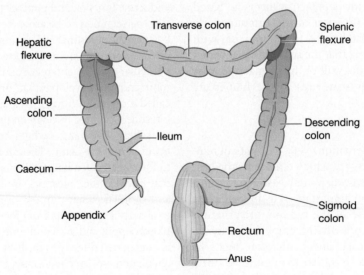

Fig. 7.4 The large intestine.

more common in affluent countries like the United States, the United Kingdom and others in Europe. With appropriate lifestyle choices, around one-quarter of colorectal cancers could be preventable. Diets high in fiber tend to decrease stool transit time and possibly limit the time any carcinogens remain in the system and are therefore associated with reduced risk of developing colon cancer. Patients with a history of benign polyps are at greater risk of developing colorectal cancer. Familial bowel cancer makes up a small percentage of cases. Generally, mortality rates are decreasing in developed countries, suggesting that treatment is becoming more effective and reflective of the success of screening programmes that have been introduced since the 1990s.

Bowel Cancer Screening

Bowel cancer survival is directly related to the stage at presentation, with early-stage detection leading to better survival rates. Screening for bowel cancer was introduced in the United States in the 1990s and the United Kingdom between 2006 and 2010. In the United Kingdom, this now takes the form of a Faecal Immunochemical Test (FIT), which replaced the guaiac Faecal Occult Blood Test around 2017–2019 and involves individuals between 50 and 75 years of age. After a positive test, the individual is invited for a colonoscopy for further investigation. Issues around uptake of the test persist. In the United Kingdom, this stands at around 65%, and although higher than the national 60% standard, it still suggests there remain barriers to taking the test. Recent studies suggest that men are less likely to take the test, and because the test is undertaken in the home environment, it often gets forgotten or other things take priority. There also remains fear of the outcome of any test or a misconception that the test is not relevant to the individual. Low health literacy and numeracy are also cited as possible barriers, and reduced uptake is seen in lower socioeconomic groups.

Screening for bowel cancer has been successful in reducing mortality. Evidence from the United States, Japan and Israel, where the screening programme is well established, point to this fact. Generally, when a screening programme is introduced, there is an initial increase in incidence reported, something already seen in the aforementioned countries and now being seen in the United Kingdom. However, evidence would suggest that this increased incidence results in many more early stage (stage I and II) cancers or, indeed, benign polyps(adenomas) being diagnosed. Removal of these polyps and subsequent follow-up will further reduce incidences of invasive bowel cancer.

Staging

Confusion may still arise over the use of the Dukes and TNM staging systems. Both systems define stage by the extent of infiltration into the mucosa and muscle and beyond and by lymph node involvement; however, whereas the Dukes system states lymph nodes are involved, the TNM will be more detailed, giving number and location of involved nodes. Both depth of invasion and lymph node involvement will have a significant bearing on prognosis.

Treatment

Surgery remains the cornerstone of treatment and can be curative for early-stage disease. Because of the vascular nature of the colon, many patients have blood-borne spread to the liver and lungs on presentation. Surgery may be used to remove small solitary metastases in the liver or lungs.

Chemotherapy will be used for patients with later stage disease and usually involves the FOLFOX (folinic acid, 5-fluorouracil, oxaliplatin) combination of drugs. Radiotherapy is seldom used for colon cancers, mainly because of the radiosensitive nature of the colon mucosa, but may be administered for cancers in the rectal area.

Around 80% or more of colon cancers will demonstrate overexpression of EGFR. EGFR-directed therapies, such as cetuximab, aflibercept or panitumumab, may be added to chemotherapy in advanced disease. A point of note: Many colon cancers may also demonstrate mutated KRAS. If this is the case, then EGFR-directed therapies are unlikely to work, and unfortunately, there appears to be no effective KRAS-directed therapy at present. Testing for EGFR positivity along with mutated KRAS is an important additional prognostic indicator. Furthermore, around 10% of colon cancers will demonstrate BRAF mutations, and this particular subset of patients tends to have more aggressive disease and may not respond as well to current chemotherapy regimens. Immunotherapy in the form of checkpoint inhibitor drugs, such as nivolumab and pembrolizumab, may also be used in the advanced stage setting.

Survival

The survival of patients with colorectal cancer is very much influenced by stage at presentation. Unfortunately, around 50% (United Kingdom) of people present with stage III (27%) or stage IV (23%) disease. Fig. 7.5 demonstrates the relationship between stage at presentation and survival.

As can be seen, the 5-year survival at stage I is around 90%, with stage II survival over 80%. Most patients with stage IV do not survive more than 5 years. The principle underpinning the bowel cancer screening programmes around the world is to diagnose more people with earlier stage cancer. As screening programmes progress, the number of patients presenting with stage I and II disease will increase.

Overcoming the barriers to this screening programme is therefore essential in improving outcome for people diagnosed with bowel cancer.

Anal Cancer

The anal canal is approximately 4 cm long and extends from the rectum to the anal orifice. The lower half is lined by squamous epithelium and the upper half by columnar epithelium. Anal cancer is an uncommon malignancy, and the main histology is SCC in the lower half, with the occasional adenocarcinoma in the upper half and some melanomas. Overall, the incidence of anal cancer is increasing. Infection with the human papilloma virus (HPV) is a known risk factor, so individuals who engage in receptive anal sex will be at higher risk of anal cancer. Higher rates of anal cancer are also found in people who smoke. The main presenting symptoms are bleeding, pain and itching, which can often be confused with those of haemorrhoids.

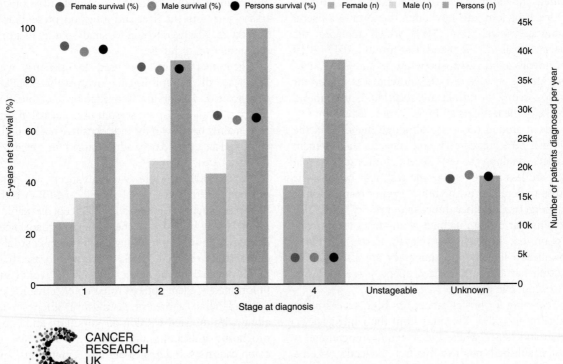

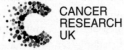

Fig. 7.5 Bowel cancer 5-year net survival by stage, with incidence by stage. *(Reproduced with permission from Cancer Research UK. https://www.cancerresearchuk.org/health-professional/cancer-statistics/statistics-by-cancer-type/bowel-cancer/survival#heading-Three. Accessed January 2022.)*

Treatment

Small tumours may be resected locally, and radio-therapy offers a good chance of cure for larger tumours. High doses of radiation may cause problems with fibrosis of the anal canal and/or sphincter in the long term. Concurrent chemotherapy in the form of 5FU and mitomycin in combination has been shown to improve survival rates in selected patients.

Liver, Pancreas and Gallbladder

The liver, pancreas and gallbladder are accessory organs of the digestive system. They produce secretions that are transported to the small intestine via a series of ducts to aid in the breakdown of foodstuffs.

Bile, produced by hepatocytes in the liver, is stored in the gallbladder. When needed, it flows to the small intestine via the common bile duct. Just before entering the duodenum, the common bile duct combines with the pancreatic duct, which brings bicarbonated pancreatic juice to the small intestine. Both join the duodenum at the hepatopancreatic ampulla (ampulla of Vater).

LIVER

The liver is the largest gland in the body and lies under the diaphragm. It extends from the right side across the midline to the stomach. The liver is divided into the right and left lobes (Fig. 7.6). The right lobe is further subdivided into the right lobe proper, the caudate

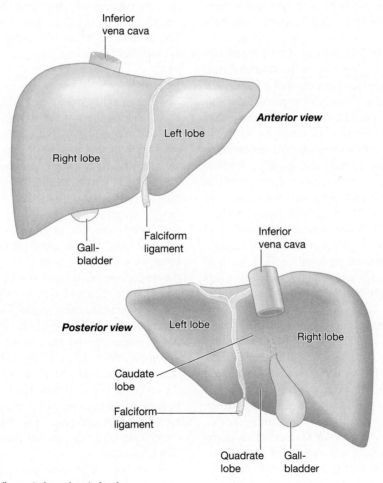

Fig. 7.6 The lobes of the liver, anterior and posterior views.

lobe and the quadrate lobe. Each lobe is divided into hepatic lobules that are roughly hexagonal in shape. Each lobule is made up of epithelial cells called hepatocytes (true liver cells) arranged in irregular columns around a central vein. Blood sinusoids, which are partly lined with stellate reticuloendothelial (Kupffer) cells, run between the columns. The Kupffer cells destroy worn-out red and white blood cells. Surrounding the liver cells are bile canaliculi, which collect bile produced by the hepatocytes and transfer it to the right and left hepatic ducts. The liver receives blood from two sources: the hepatic artery (a direct branch of the aorta) and the hepatic portal vein, which carries blood rich in nutrients, toxins and possibly drugs from the digestive tract. This blood is conveyed to the lobules and the nutrients and oxygen are taken up by the hepatocytes. The hepatocytes in turn secrete their products, which may be needed by other cells, back into the blood. Each lobule is supplied with an abundance of blood, making the liver an extremely vascular organ. Because all the blood from the digestive tract goes first to the liver, it is a common site for metastases.

Primary liver cancer, known as hepatocellular carcinoma (HCC), is very rare but, if found early, may be cured by surgical resection. However, metastases to the liver remain the most common tumour found in the liver. Hepatoblastoma may also occur in children. Cirrhosis of the liver due to excessive alcohol intake is the greatest risk factor and even greater if accompanied by heavy smoking. Other major risk factors include hepatitis B and C. Aflatoxins, found on the surface of mouldy nuts and beans, are another known carcinogen, and populations that eat much of these kinds of foods, such as in Africa and Asia, see increased levels of HCC. In some rare instances, HCC can be seen to run in families.

Typical symptoms will include unexplained weight loss and abdominal swelling and may be due to ascites and jaundice. Raised alfa-fetoprotein levels can indicate the presence of HCC and can be used as a tumour marker. Most people who present will be men over the age of 60 years, and the United Kingdom has seen an increase in incidence over the last 30 years.

The TNM staging system for liver cancer is determined by the presence of solitary or multiple tumours and whether there is evidence of vascular invasion. Furthermore, stage may be influenced by the general

health and condition of the patient along with the level of liver function. All these factors, along with the amount of cirrhosis present, will be considered in decisions around treatment. Small solitary tumours may be removed or radiofrequency ablation can be attempted. Unfortunately, many patients will present with multifocal disease, making surgical cure difficult to achieve. However, surgery still offers the main chance of cure. Embolisation may be a strategy to starve the tumour of blood and limit potential metastases. Furthermore, antiangiogenic drugs such as sorafenib and lenvatinib, or checkpoint inhibitor drugs such as nivolumab may be used for advanced disease.

Survival is very much influenced by the stage at presentation along with the age and condition of the presenting patient. Unfortunately, many will present as older patients with low liver function and at a late stage, which means that survival in this group is very low. In cases where disease is diagnosed early, survival is much better.

PANCREAS

The pancreas (Fig. 7.7) lies behind the stomach in the C-shaped loop of the duodenum in direct contact with the stomach and spleen. Major blood vessels, such as the mesenteric artery and veins, pass close to the body of the pancreas. Microscopically, the pancreas is composed of a large number of lobules surrounded by fatty tissue. Each lobule is composed of glandular epithelium lined with many specialised cells that produce pancreatic secretions. Of these cells, 1% are called pancreatic islets and the other 99% are acinic cells. The pancreatic islets are the endocrine portion of the pancreas and secrete glucagon, insulin and somatostatin. The acinic cells secrete pancreatic juice to aid the digestive process. Pancreatic juice is secreted into the pancreatic duct, which transports the juice to the duodenum via the hepatopancreatic ampulla (ampulla of Vater). Shortly before this ampulla, the pancreatic duct is joined by the common bile duct from the liver and gallbladder. Because of the proximity of so many organs, it is common for a pancreatic cancer to invade one or more of these structures. This makes pancreatic cancer very difficult to cure.

Pancreatic cancer ranks as the 10th most common cancer in the United Kingdom and 11th in the United

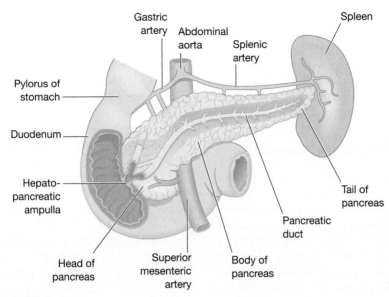

Fig. 7.7 Relational anatomy of the pancreas.

States. Because of the poor prognosis associated with the disease, pancreatic cancer constitutes a significant health risk. Men are more likely to get the disease, although the male-to-female ratio is becoming more even, and this is possibly reflective of the risk factors associated with pancreatic cancer, with heavy smoking being the greatest. Most cases will occur over the age of 70 years, and it is very uncommon below 40 years. Obesity is also a known risk factor, and around 5% will be related to hereditary disease, such as those carrying a faulty BRCA2 gene. Mortality rates tend to mirror the incidence rates, with patients rarely surviving a year. Most pancreatic tumours are of ductal type (adenocarcinomas), starting in the cells that line the ductal network throughout the pancreas.

Typical signs and symptoms of pancreatic cancer include jaundice, abdominal or lower back pain and unexplained weight loss. Light-coloured stools, dark urine and loss of appetite are also common. Around 50% of patients will have diabetes, but as pancreatic cancer itself can cause diabetes, it is sometimes difficult to say whether this caused the disease or is a result of the disease. Unfortunately, these symptoms will not be obvious until the disease is at an advanced stage, with early-stage disease being difficult to detect because it exhibits no real symptoms.

Staging for pancreatic cancer is based on the size of the tumour, with small (<2 cm) tumours being stage I. Involvement of other structures and lymph node involvement indicate later stage disease. Around 85% of tumours will arise in the head of the pancreas, 15% in the body and 5% in the tail. Because of the relationship of the pancreas with many surrounding structures, it is not uncommon for this disease to locally infiltrate said organs; and involvement of the duodenum, stomach and transverse colon is common, and peritoneal involvement is seen in many patients. Survival for patients with pancreatic cancer is poor, with surgery offering the best chance of disease-free survival. Chemotherapy, 5FU or gemcitabine may be offered post-surgically.

GALLBLADDER

The gallbladder is a pear-shaped organ that lies on the undersurface of the liver. Its function is to store bile and secrete it into the duodenum via the common bile duct when influenced by the amount of fat in the intestine. Bile is an emulsifier; that is, it breaks down fat for the body to process it more easily. Gallbladder cancer is uncommon and tends to be associated with gallstones. Many patients are found to have cancer on routine removal of the gallbladder as a remedy for gallstones. This leads to cure with no further treatment required. Most tumours of the gallbladder are adenocarcinomas of various subtypes: Signet ring cell, clear cell, colloid, small (oat) cell and others are locally invasive to the liver and bile duct. Gallbladder cancer that has penetrated the muscularis and serosa is curable in fewer than 5% of patients.

Carcinoid (Neuroendocrine) Tumours

Carcinoid or neuroendocrine tumours can arise in various places throughout the body but most commonly in the digestive tract. They occur in enteroendocrine cells that are dispersed throughout the stomach and small and large intestines. This network of specialised cells plays a role in stimulating the organs of the digestive system to generate secretions that aid the digestive process. Serotonin is released by neuroendocrine cells within the digestive tract in response to distension of the intestine by food. The serotonin will then stimulate the muscle of the intestine to contract, thus stimulating peristalsis and movement of food along the intestine. If too much serotonin is released, which may be the case in carcinoid tumours, muscle contraction in the gut will increase, leading to faster transit times and diarrhoea. Carcinoid tumours are classified as neuroendocrine tumours and are often asymptomatic, mainly because of their slow-growing nature. They can occur anywhere where enteroendocrine cells are found, but the most common sites are the appendix, small bowel and rectum. Patients with carcinoid tumours may present with carcinoid syndrome, typically with flushing, diarrhoea and abdominal cramps. Carcinoid syndrome is caused by oversecretion of serotonin by the affected cells. Surgical removal of the affected site offers a good chance of cure for localised disease. Radiotherapy and chemotherapy are largely ineffective.

SELF-ASSESSMENT QUESTIONS

Answer true or false to the following. Answers are on page 165–166.

1 The pancreas, gallbladder and liver are termed accessory organs of the digestive system.

2 The oesophagus is lined entirely with squamous epithelium.

3 Smoking and drinking are main causative factors for squamous cell carcinoma of the oesophagus.

4 Staging of oesophageal cancer is based on the level of infiltration through the muscle layer of the oesophagus.

5 Barrett oesophagus increases the risk of cancer of the oesophagus.

6 The stomach is lined with glandular epithelium.

7 Squamous cell carcinoma is the predominant tumour of the stomach.

8 Some stomach tumours may be described as HER2+ve.

9 The order of sections of the small intestine (in the direction of the digestive process) is ileum, jejunum, duodenum.

10 The lining of the small intestine includes aggregated lymphatic tissue (Peyer patches).

11 Squamous cell carcinoma is the most common type of tumour in the small intestine.

12 Adenocarcinomas make up about 90% of cases of colorectal cancer.

13 Colorectal cancer is associated with a high-fibre diet.

14 The staging of colorectal cancer is based on the level of infiltration of the muscle layer.

15 Patients with mutated KRAS are often given cetuximab alongside chemotherapy for late-stage disease.

16 *Infection with HPV is a known risk factor in anal cancer.*

17 *Metastases are the most common primary liver tumour.*

18 *The pancreas is both an endocrine gland and an exocrine gland.*

19 *Staging for pancreatic cancer is based on the size of the tumour.*

20 *Carcinoid tumours arise from the enteroendocrine cells of the gastrointestinal tract.*

Urinary System Tumours

Chapter Outline

Objectives

By the end of this chapter, the reader should be able to:

- Outline the anatomy and histology of the kidneys and relate this to the different types of cancer.
- Summarise the risk factors associated with kidney cancer and describe the most common signs and symptoms.
- Understand the role of standard and targeted treatments for kidney cancer.
- Describe the anatomy of the urinary bladder.
- Demonstrate an understanding of the staging for bladder cancer and how this relates to the management of patients with bladder cancer.

The urinary system consists of two kidneys, two ureters, one urinary bladder and one urethra.

The Kidneys and Ureters

The kidneys are situated behind the peritoneum (retroperitoneal) on the posterior abdominal wall (Fig. 8.1). They are approximately 9 cm long and 6 cm wide and are oriented so that the upper lobe is closer to midline. Normal kidneys have a shiny, reddish-brown appearance. Their function is to regulate the volume and composition of blood in the body by removing waste materials. They cleanse the plasma and adjust the salt and pH content. The resultant waste product is called urine. Adults normally excrete 1 to 1.5 L of urine per day. Once produced, the urine is conveyed via the ureters to the urinary bladder, where it is stored prior to excretion via the urethra.

The kidney is divided into an outer cortex and inner medulla section (Fig. 8.2). Within the medulla are 5 to 14 striated triangular structures called renal pyramids. The cortex extends between these pyramids, forming renal columns. The cortex and the

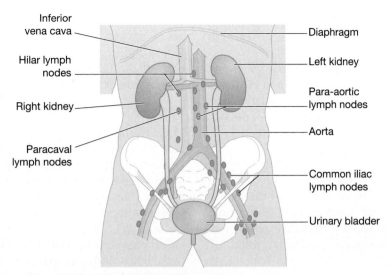

Fig. 8.1 Relational anatomy of the kidneys, showing regional lymphatic drainage.

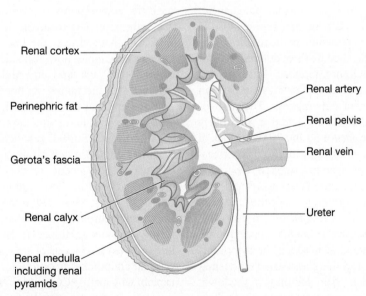

Fig. 8.2 Coronal section through the kidney.

pyramids constitute the renal parenchyma; that is, the functional part of the kidney. The renal parenchyma consists of millions of nephrons with their associated collecting ducts and blood supply. The nephrons filter the blood and ultimately produce the urine.

The urine is conveyed via the collecting tubules into the central part of the kidney, called the renal pelvis, which is typically whitish grey in appearance.

Interestingly, the cells lining the renal pelvis are transitional epithelial cells. The difference in the functions of the renal parenchyma and the renal pelvis results in different malignant histologies (see below). The kidney parenchyma is surrounded by a tough renal capsule, which itself is enveloped by a layer of fatty tissue called perinephric fat. Between the kidney, the psoas muscle and the lumbar spine is a band of connective tissue referred to as Gerota fascia, an important landmark when considering advanced stages of renal cell carcinoma (RCC).

Lymphatically, the kidneys drain into the lymph nodes medial to the hilum (renal hilar) and the nodes surrounding the aorta (para-aortic) and inferior vena cava (paracaval). All regional lymph nodes of the kidney are retroperitoneal.

ONCOLOGY

Carcinoma of the kidney accounts for approximately 2% of all cancers. Of these, 90% are of the kidney parenchyma (renal cell carcinomas or RCCs) and 15% are of the renal pelvis (transitional cell carcinomas), reflective of the change in epithelium within the kidney.

Renal Cell Carcinoma

RCCs are the most common of the renal malignancies and also known as adenocarcinomas, as they arise in the modified glandular epithelium of the tubules of the nephron. Pathologically, they are three different types – clear cell, papillary and chromophobe – and are distinct histologies, and correct evaluation may have an impact on likely treatment and prognosis. The male-to-female ratio is approximately 2:1, and it is most likely to present between the ages of 60 and 70 years. Risk of RCC is increased with smoking, with the risk increasing with the number of cigarettes smoked. Obesity is another known risk factor and may be associated with up to 50% of all RCCs. Furthermore, alcohol and high blood pressure are cited as risk factors, and a small percentage of cases will have a hereditary background.

The body is very good at masking the symptoms associated with RCC, and the 'classic triad' of haematuria (blood in the urine), pain and mass in the lower flank area of the body is, more often than not, indicative of late-stage disease. Other symptoms may include fever, and some patients will be diagnosed incidentally when being investigated for other ailments.

Staging

Staging of RCC is based on the degree of spread within and, more importantly, beyond the kidney. Invasion beyond Gerota fascia would be the difference between stage III and stage IV disease, for example. Although involvement of blood vessels, such as the vena cava, is generally associated with poor prognosis, this may not be the case for disease otherwise confined to the kidney. RCCs have a tendency to metastasise to other parts of the body, principally lung, mainly via the bloodstream rather than lymphatically.

Treatment

The mainstay of treatment for kidney cancer is surgery. Early-stage disease is often treated with radical nephrectomy that will include removal of the kidney, adrenal gland, perirenal fat and Gerota fascia, with or without a regional lymph node dissection. For selected patients with a small tumour confined to the kidney, partial nephrectomy may be an option. External beam radiotherapy can be used, both pre- and postoperatively, but is often only palliative. Patients with later stage disease may benefit from embolisation of the tumour but, again, this is generally seen as a palliative measure, and response to cytotoxic chemotherapy is generally poor. The treatment horizon for metastatic RCC has changed over the last 20 years, with more biological therapies now available (Fig. 8.3).

Interferon alfa and interleukin-2 are cytokines involved in promoting a nonspecific, generalised immune effect in the body. Such drugs were used as part of an immunotherapy approach to dealing with advanced RCC. Further research into the biology of RCC has demonstrated an association with both an enhanced angiogenetic tendency and an aberrant growth pathway in these tumours, particularly clear cell RCC. Most clear cell tumours demonstrate an alteration in chromosome 3p that in turn leads to inactivation of the von Hippel Lindau (VHL) gene, which leads to increased levels of angiogenic factors such as vascular endothelial growth factor (VEGF). This might explain why many RCCs tend to be extremely vascular in nature. Antiangiogenic drugs, such as bevacizumab (Avastin), sorafenib (Nexavar) and, more recently, axitinib (Inlyta), have become an integral part of treatment in this advanced setting. RCCs also demonstrate aberrations in the P13K/mToR signalling pathway and everolimus (Afinitor); an mToR inhibitor is an alternative if the antiangiogenic drugs do not work. More recently, checkpoint inhibitor drugs, such as nivolumab (Opdivo), have shown to be effective and may be used as an alternative if the previous drugs are intolerable to the patients or do not work.

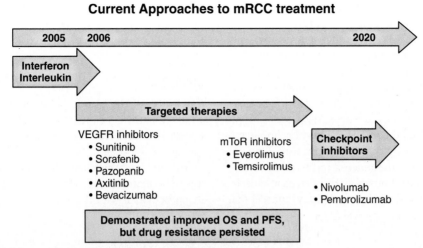

Fig. 8.3 Targeted approach to treatment for metastatic renal cell carcinoma.

Prognosis is directly related to the stage or degree of tumour dissemination. RCC confined to the kidney and surrounding area is often curable. Although some patients with regional lymphatic involvement achieve prolonged survival, involvement of lymphatic groups and the presence of distant metastases are associated with poor prognosis.

Renal Pelvis Tumours

Because of the anatomical relationship between the renal pelvis and ureter, it is useful to consider these two sites together. Histologically, the two share the same basic type of epithelial lining, namely transitional cell epithelium or urothelium. The majority of renal pelvis and ureteric tumours are transitional cell carcinomas, with the occasional squamous cell carcinoma presenting. These tumours account for only a small percentage of kidney tumours and tend to be curable if diagnosed early enough. Some of the tumours that present are multifocal in origin, and the treatment is therefore designed to take this into account. Where multifocal disease of the renal pelvis and ureters is present, the probability of bladder involvement increases significantly.

Staging

The staging of these tumours is very similar to that of bladder cancer (see later) in that the important characteristic is the depth of invasion of the tumour in the renal pelvis or ureter.

Treatment

Treatment for these tumours consists primarily of surgery. Generally, unless highly localised disease can be proved, total nephroureterectomy with removal of the bladder cuff is necessary. In selected patients, partial removal can be undertaken.

Patients presenting with superficial tumours have a high percentage chance of cure (approximately 90%). Of those patients with more deeply invasive disease, there is a 10% to 15% likelihood of cure; however, if the ureteric wall has been breached and/or there are metastases present, the likelihood of cure is very poor.

The Urinary Bladder

The urinary bladder is a reservoir for urine. It is a hollow muscular organ situated behind the symphysis pubis. In the male, the bladder is separated from the rectum (which lies behind) by the rectovesical fascia, which contains the seminal vesicles and vas deferens. Below the bladder is the prostate gland, which encloses the first part of the urethra. In the female, the bladder lies in front of the vagina and the uterus, which also extends over the top of the bladder. The uterus and bladder are separated by a fold of peritoneum called the uterovesical pouch. The relational anatomy is shown in more detail in Fig. 8.4A and B.

The bladder consists of an inner mucosa, typically transitional cell epithelium, or urothelium, which is generally in folds known as rugae. A triangular area known as the trigone is easily identifiable by the two ureters that enter the bladder and the urethra that leaves it at the bladder neck. This area is typically smoother than the rest of the bladder lining and dips slightly in the ureter-urethra direction. The submucosa helps attach the mucosa to the thick muscle layer of the bladder known as the detrusor muscle. This is made up of smooth (involuntary) muscle that

contracts the bladder when expelling urine. A final outer layer that covers only the superior portion of the bladder is sometimes referred to as the serosa or adventitia (Fig. 8.5).

ONCOLOGY

Carcinoma of the bladder accounts for 3% to 4% of all malignancies. The male-to-female ratio is approximately 4:1, and the disease usually occurs between the ages of 55 and 80 years. Although generally unknown, the cause may be linked to certain factors. The increase in environmental carcinogens and, in particular, 2-naphthylamine in the production of

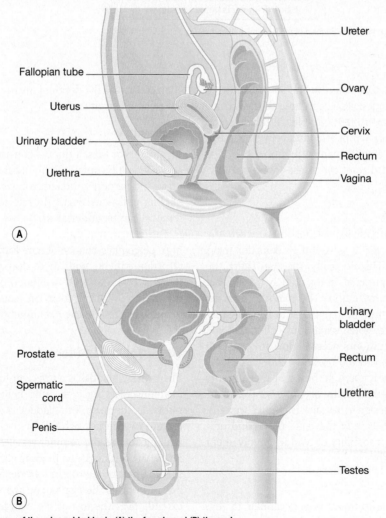

Fig. 8.4 Relational anatomy of the urinary bladder in (A) the female and (B) the male.

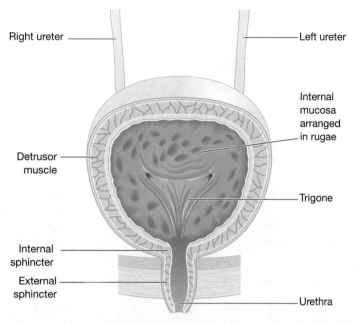

Right ureter

Left ureter

Internal mucosa arranged in rugae

Detrusor muscle

Trigone

Internal sphincter

External sphincter

Urethra

Fig. 8.5 The urinary bladder.

aniline dyes is a known risk factor. Smokers are also six times more likely to develop bladder cancer. The majority of cancers of the bladder are transitional cell (urothelial) carcinomas, with some adenocarcinomas and lymphomas occurring. Squamous cell carcinoma is rare in the UK but can occur as a result of exposure to schistosoma, parasitic worms common in Egypt and central Africa.

Macroscopically, the disease can be divided into superficial (often referred to as papillary) carcinoma and solid carcinoma, which tends to be nodular in appearance and more infiltrative. Papillary tumours have narrow stalks and project into the lumen of the bladder. If they are confined to the surface of the epithelium, they are described as noninvasive, but once the submucosa is involved, the tumour is frankly invasive. Solid or sessile tumours appear as flat lesions confined to the mucosal lining of the bladder and are described as carcinomas in situ (Fig. 8.6).

Staging

Stage will be determined following an initial transurethral resection of the bladder tumour (TURBT). As previously described, the staging of bladder cancer is strongly related to the depth of invasion into the

muscle of the bladder wall of the tumour (Fig. 8.7) and has a marked effect on the management of the disease. Often, tumours present with multifocal origin, and this must be considered in deciding on the treatment regimen.

Treatment

Treatment for carcinoma of the bladder is strongly related to the stage of the disease and will often consist of surgery, radiotherapy and chemotherapy in combination or alone.

Superficial tumours are removed by transurethral resection (TUR) or diathermy (fulguration). External beam radiotherapy is rarely used in these cases because of the high chance of recurrence. Regular cystoscopy follow-up, with or without TUR/diathermy, can be very successful. For recurrence or multifocal disease, chemotherapy with mitomycin C is effective, or immunotherapy with BCG (bacillus Calmette-Guérin) can be used as an alternative. These drugs tend to be given intravesically – that is, they are introduced into the bladder lumen via a urethral catheter.

For invasive tumours with no evidence of metastasis (stage II), radical cystectomy may be offered, with patients unfit for this procedure given radiotherapy.

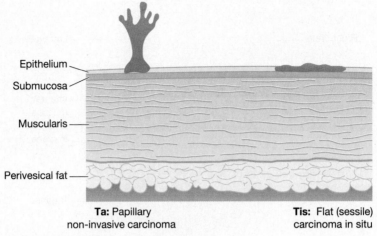

Epithelium
Submucosa
Muscularis
Perivesical fat

Ta: Papillary
non-invasive carcinoma

Tis: Flat (sessile)
carcinoma in situ

Fig. 8.6 Superficial and invasive tumours of the bladder.

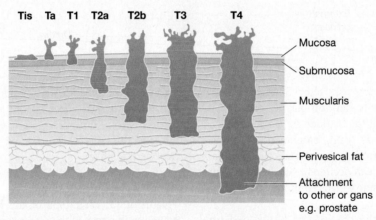

Tis   Ta   T1   T2a   T2b   T3   T4

Mucosa
Submucosa
Muscularis
Perivesical fat
Attachment
to other or gans
e.g. prostate

Fig. 8.7 Staging of bladder cancer is based on the depth of invasion through the bladder wall.

For patients with stage III or IV[a] disease, chemotherapy with or without radiotherapy will be an option. Patients with demonstrable metastases will be given chemotherapy. Typical chemotherapy drugs used will be methotrexate, vinblastine, doxorubicin, cisplatin (MVAC) or gemcitabine with cisplatin.

Adenocarcinomas and squamous cell carcinomas of the bladder tend to be insensitive to radiotherapy and therefore the treatment of choice is surgery.

Prognosis is related to the depth of invasion of the tumour; patients with superficial tumours can survive many years with regular follow-up.

---

[a]Stage IVb bladder cancer can be a tumour that has invaded the pelvic or abdominal wall but investigations have failed to demonstrate lymphatic or wider disease.

SELF-ASSESSMENT QUESTIONS

Answer true or false to the following. Answers are on page 165–166.

1 *Adults normally excrete 1 to 1.5 L of urine per day.*

2 *The kidneys are divided into an outer medulla and inner cortex.*

3 *Epithelial cells line the tubules of the nephron.*

4 *RCC is the most common type of kidney tumour.*

5 *RCC predominantly arises in the proximal convoluted tubule of the kidney.*

6 *Invasion beyond Gerota fascia would indicate stage IV disease.*

7 *External beam radiotherapy plays a major role in the radical treatment of RCC.*

8 *Angiogenic inhibitor drugs play an important role in metastatic RCC.*

9 *Renal pelvic tumours are mainly transitional cell carcinomas.*

10 *The renal pelvis has the same epithelial lining as the ureter.*

11 *Staging of renal pelvis and ureteric tumours is based on the size of the tumour.*

12 *Total nephroureterectomy and removal of the bladder cuff is the mainstay of treatment for renal pelvis and ureteric tumours.*

13 *The urinary bladder produces urine.*

14 *The urinary bladder is lined with transitional cell epithelium.*

15 *Most bladder cancer occurs in women between the ages of 55 and 80 years.*

16 *Papillary carcinoma is suggestive of invasion into the wall of the bladder.*

17 *Squamous cell carcinoma is the most common malignancy of the bladder.*

18 *Treatment of carcinoma of the bladder is related to the depth of invasion of the tumour through the bladder wall.*

19 *A T3 bladder cancer invades through the perivesical fat.*

20 *Mitomycin is a drug often used to treat multifocal bladder cancer.*

The Male Reproductive System

Chapter Outline

Objectives

By the end of this chapter, the reader should be able to:

- Outline the anatomy of the testes and prostate and relate this to the signs and symptoms associated with cancers in these areas.
- Summarise the risk factors associated with cancers of the testes and prostate.
- Explain the role of tumour markers in the diagnosis and treatment of cancers of the testes and prostate.
- Explain the difference between seminoma and nonseminoma of the testes.
- Understand the role of surgery, radiotherapy, chemotherapy and hormone therapy in the treatment of male cancers.

The male reproductive system (Fig. 9.1) is composed of organs that are concerned with the production, maturation and transfer of mature sperm. Production is initiated in the testes, and the resulting sperm are transferred from the testes via a duct system where the sperm gradually mature and are stored until ejaculation. Accessory reproductive glands produce most of the fluid or semen that transports and nourishes the sperm, and these include the seminal vesicles, bulbourethral glands and the prostate gland.

The Testes

The testes (Fig. 9.2) are a pair of small oval organs about 5 cm in length and weighing 10 to 15 g. They develop high on the posterior wall of the abdomen at the level of the kidney. Toward the end, the seventh month of foetal development, the testes usually descend into the pelvic cavity, through the peritoneum and through a small inguinal opening or canal, out of the body and into the scrotum. As

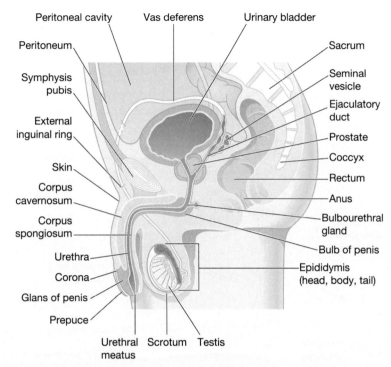

Fig. 9.1 Relational anatomy of the male reproductive system.

the testes pass through the abdomen, they bring with them their own connective tissue composed of a cremaster muscle; blood, lymph and nerve supply; and the vas deferens. These structures are known collectively as the spermatic cord and hold the testes suspended in the scrotal sac. As the testes pass through the inguinal canal, they acquire peritoneal coverings: a thin outer serous layer called the tunica vaginalis (which also lines the inner scrotal sacs) and a thicker fibrous white inner layer called the tunica albuginea that also extends into the mass of the testicular tissue and divides it into 200 to 300 compartments called lobules (see Fig. 9.2). Each of these lobules contains:

- Specialised interstitial cells called Leydig cells (which secrete male hormones or androgens, especially testosterone) and Sertoli cells that regulate metabolism and provide support and nourishment of the developing sperm
- Seminiferous tubules – within each lobule are between one and four small coiled seminiferous tubules where sperm production is initiated (spermatogenesis).

Luteinising hormone (LH) and follicle-stimulating hormone (FSH), both secreted by the pituitary gland, are essential in spermatogenesis. LH stimulates the Leydig cells to secrete testosterone. Testosterone is the male hormone responsible for secondary male sex characteristics and also stimulates the Sertoli cells, which are also targeted by FSH. Sertoli cells are responsible for nourishing and supporting the development of sperm within the seminiferous tubules.

The seminiferous tubules from each lobule join to form a plexus of vessels called the rete (pronounced ree-tee) testis; these drain into a series of sperm ducts called the efferent ducts, which pierce the tunica vaginalis and converge to become the head of the epididymis. The epididymis is a tightly coiled tube encased in a fibrous layer; it is comma-shaped and lies superior and posterior to the testis. The epididymis is composed of a head, body and tail that are continuous with the vas deferens. The epididymis acts as a duct through which sperm pass, but it also stores the sperm for 1 to 3 weeks while they mature, and it secretes a small part of the seminal fluid (semen). The developing young

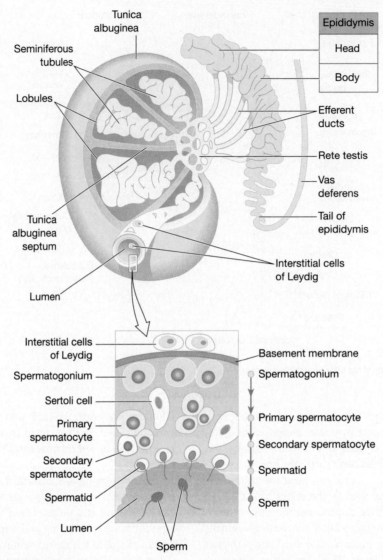

Fig. 9.2 Anatomy of the testis and scrotum.

sperm (spermatozoa) require a cooler temperature than the rest of the body, and two muscles assist this process: the smooth dartos muscle from the scrotum, which causes the scrotal skin to wrinkle, and the cremaster muscle, which lies in the spermatic cord and allows the testes to rise or fall to maintain the temperature at 3°C below core body temperature.

The descent of the testes into the scrotum is critically important for sperm production; failure of this to happen is known as cryptorchidism (hidden testes

or maldescent). Whilst most maldescended testes will spontaneously descend during the first year of life, intervention in the form of orchidopexy is necessary if this does not occur. A history of cryptorchidism is a strong risk factor for developing testicular cancer.

It is important to note that because the testes originate high on the upper abdominal wall, the subsequent lymphatic drainage differs from that of the surrounding scrotum. Thus, the testis, because of its original embryonic site of origin in the abdomen, initially drains along the spermatic cord and then up to the lymph nodes around the aorta and inferior vena.

The scrotal sac, however, drains first to regional nodes and then into inguinal nodes, so a surgical procedure to access the testes through the scrotal sac (transscrotal orchidectomy) is not advised. The preferred access is through a high incision in the inguinal area to prevent the risk of scrotal recurrence or later inguinal node involvement.

ONCOLOGY

Testicular cancer is the most common solid tumour among young men aged 15 to 39 years. Around 9000 new cases are reported each year in the United States and around 2000 in the United Kingdom. It is more common in White males, although the reasons for this are largely unknown, and it is most common between the ages of 15 and 40 years. Treatment and, consequently, survival of testicular cancer has been one of the success stories of modern cancer treatments. Survival rates in excess of 95% are seen and are due in part to a better understanding of the types of testicular cancer, the ability to monitor various tumour markers and the administration of platinum-based chemotherapy drugs.

HISTOLOGY

Referring back to the internal structure of the testes (see Fig. 9.2), it can be seen that they are composed mainly of two types of cells. There are the supportive cells that help with the maturation of sperm, such as the Leydig (interstitial) and Sertoli (nurse) cells, and the germ cells that will produce the sperm itself. Germ cells are primitive cells that are found in the developing embryo and will eventually mature to become all of the tissues of the human body. However, some germ cells remain as germ cells and will migrate to the testes in the male and ovaries in the female. These resident germ cells retain the ability to produce all of the tissues of the body, an important consideration when thinking about the pathological presentation of some of these tumours. The great majority of testicular tumours (90% to 95%) are germ cell tumours (GCTs). These GCTs are classified into two groups, seminomas and nonseminomas, along with other non-GCTs (Box 9.1). Non-GCTs consisting of rare tumours affect the supporting cells as mentioned above.

BOX 9.1 TYPES OF TESTICULAR TUMOURS

Germ Cell		Non-Germ Cell
Seminoma	Nonseminoma • Embryonal • Teratoma • Choriocarcinoma • Yolk sac	• Leydig tumours • Sertoli cell tumours

All GCTs arise from the germ cells found inside the seminiferous tubules and will often secrete specialised proteins, such as alfa-fetoprotein (AFP) and human chorionic gonadotropin (hCG), that are normally produced by germ cells in the developing foetus (see Chapter 1). AFP and hCG can be used as tumour markers, as they are useful in monitoring how well the patient's tumour responds to any therapy.

Seminomas are the most common type of GCT and arise from the germ cells that continue to divide uncontrollably without differentiating (maturing) into other types of cells. Pathologically, they are said to have a 'fried egg' appearance (larger, with a central nucleus and clear cytoplasm) and will group together to form lobules surrounded by fibrous tissue, which will form a kind of capsule that separates the tumour from normal tissue. It is often infiltrated by lymphocytes. Importantly, seminomas may also secrete placental alkaline phosphatase (PLAP), an enzyme normally secreted by the placenta, and raised levels could indicate malignancy. Seminomas tend to spread more readily via the lymphatic system; therefore, investigation of the regional lymphatics within the abdomen (as described earlier) will be warranted and help in the staging and possible management of these patients.

Nonseminomas tend to be more common in younger men (in their 20s) and constitute approximately 40% of all testicular cancers. In 90% of nonseminomas, a tumour marker is secreted that is very useful in monitoring therapy. They tend to be more aggressive in nature and will often metastasise via the blood. There are four classifications of nonseminoma:

• *Embryonal carcinoma* – Often, these tumours are very small, even when advanced. Microscopically, the tumours will have sections containing bleeding and often necrosis. These tumours tend to be highly infiltrative and have a high potential for metastasis.

- *Teratomas* – The name derives from the presence of different mature tissue types in the tumour (*tera-*, monster and *-oma*, tumour). *Mature cystic teratoma*, as the name suggests, is made up of cystic-like structures comprising mature tissue that may contain fully formed hair, teeth and eyes, amongst other things. These tend to be classified as benign in children but malignant in adults. *Immature teratoma* tends to occur in adults and will contain remnants of immature embryonic tissue.
- *Choriocarcinoma* derives from cells that form the placenta, most notably syncytiotrophoblasts and cytotrophoblasts. Syncytiotrophoblasts are responsible for secreting hCG; therefore, this can be raised and used in the diagnosis and management of this type of tumour. It tends to be an aggressive type of GCT in adults, locally invasive, fast growing and often producing widespread metastases and lymphatic spread.
- *Yolk sac tumours* account for most testicular tumours found in children under 15 years. In its purest form, a yolk sac tumour tends to be very aggressive and is highly likely to metastasise to the liver. Yolk sac tumours produce raised levels of AFP, which can be used to monitor response to treatment and the status of disease.

Non-GCTs derive from the supporting cells within the testes. As described earlier, these are the Sertoli cells found inside the seminiferous tubules and the Leydig cells found outside the seminiferous tubules.

- *Sertoli cell* tumours originate inside the seminiferous tubules and derive from those cells within the tubules that support the development of sperm. Such tumours tend to be small, very well differentiated and often classified as benign. They do not secrete any tumour markers.
- *Leydig tumours* originate outside the seminiferous tubules. Leydig cells secrete sex hormones, and both testosterone and oestrogen can be elevated with these tumours. Excess testosterone in children might lead to precocious puberty. Excess oestrogen may lead to delayed puberty and feminisation in young boys. In the adult, it may lead to gynaecomastia (breast enlargement), testicular atrophy, loss of libido and erectile dysfunction. Microscopically, the presence of Reinke crystals (rods of excess proteins in the cytoplasm of the cells) will help determine diagnosis.

Tumours consisting of two or more cell types make up the rest. The characteristics of various types of testicular tumours are summarised in Table 9.1.

AETIOLOGY

A history of cryptorchidism (maldescended testes) is the most important risk factor and is present in 10% of all testicular cancers. The location where the developing testicle lodges in the abdomen can affect the risk

TABLE 9.1 Characteristics of Different Types of Testicular Cancer							
	Seminoma	Embryonal	Teratoma	Choriocarcinoma	Yolk Sac	Sertoli Cell	Leydig Cell
Potential for metastasis	Low	Medium	Low	High	High	Low	Low
Route of spread	Lymphatic	Blood	Lymphatic	Blood	Blood	–	–
AFP	– –	+	–	–	++	–	–
hCG	rarely	maybe	–	+++	–	–	–
PLAP	+	–	–	–	–	–	–
Chemosensitive	+	+	Less	+++	++	–	–
Radiosensitive	+++	Less	Less	Less	Less	–	–

AFP, Alfa-fetoprotein; *hCG*, human chorionic gonadotropin; *PLAP*, placental alkaline phosphatase.

of developing cancer, as an abdominal cryptorchid testicle (where the maldescended testis may be stuck inside the abdominal cavity) is more likely to develop cancer than an inguinal testicle. Risk is increased with Klinefelter syndrome, which is typically small undeveloped testicles. In utero exposure to certain chemicals may also increase risk. Interestingly, testicular cancer is more common in White males, and many testicular cancers exhibit mutations within chromosome 12.

Clinical Features

The usual initial finding is heaviness or a painless lump in or on the testis or a change in texture of the testicular tissue, such as hardness, or the testis may become enlarged. Less commonly, there is associated pain and tenderness. Other symptoms, such as haemoptysis, back pain and loin pain or neck lymphadenopathy, unfortunately suggest widespread metastatic disease, and about 10% of patients may present with one or more of these symptoms. A relatively large proportion of patients with occult metastatic disease may not display any of these sinister symptoms at the time of diagnosis. AFP and hCG levels in the blood can be raised, indicating the presence of an active GCT. Most testicular cancer is diagnosed through self-examination, a process whereby the male regularly examines the testes for any signs of abnormality. Testicular self-examination is best attended to directly after a hot bath or shower when the muscles are at their most relaxed. This allows the individual to become familiar with the normal texture of the testes and therefore any changes can be detected at a very early stage. This form of testicular screening is cheap, noninvasive and easily reproducible, and educating young men to do this is an important part of any health education strategy.

If cancer is suspected, biochemical tests for tumour markers can show very high levels of AFP and hCG; preoperative and postoperative measurements are helpful not only in diagnosis but in staging and monitoring the response of the tumour to treatment. Serum PLAP is often raised in seminoma but not diagnostic, as it may be raised for other reasons, such as smoking. Although a clinician can palpate the testis, and ultrasound is useful to determine if the patient has testicular cancer, it is only after an inguinal orchidectomy that the testis can be directly seen and biopsies taken,

if necessary. Therefore, diagnosis is only confirmed on biopsy. Often, a chest x-ray is done to exclude the possibility of lung metastases, and a computed tomography (CT) scan is done to try and assess any local spread and possible lymphatic involvement; these evaluations are essential for correctly staging the disease and deciding the appropriate treatment.

Staging

Staging of testicular cancer is largely independent of the tumour type, although the type will influence potential treatments. An important characteristic of the TNM staging system is whether the tumour is confined to the testes or not. Invasion beyond the tunica vaginalis (outer layer) is the main difference between pT1 and pT2; vascular and/or lymphatic involvement will also influence this. Involvement of lymph nodes will indicate a later stage of disease, and as the testes descend from the posterior wall of the abdomen, they take their blood and lymphatic drainage from the area of origin so that any involvement of the lymphatic system will spread directly to the para-aortic lymph node chain that lies alongside the vertebral column at the level of the kidneys. Involvement of nodes, such as the internal and external iliac nodes, suggests that there may be local extension from the tumour involving other structures. Blood-borne metastasis, maybe to the lungs, is not uncommon, and although it would constitute late-stage disease, still remains a curable outcome for many. Serum tumour markers, as described above, also play an important part in the TNM system, with very high levels usually indicating a widespread disease.

TREATMENT OF TESTICULAR CANCER

Testicular cancer is extremely treatable and is very curable, particularly in young and middle-aged men. Management is based on whether the tumour is of seminoma or nonseminoma type and is related to the tumour's manner of spread, as seminomas tend to spread more readily via the lymphatics and nonseminomas via the blood. Seminomas are also much more sensitive to radiation and respond well to radiotherapy treatment, unlike nonseminomas (see Table 9.1). When all stages of seminoma are combined, the cure rate is over 90%; if treated at an early stage, the cure rate is almost 100%.

All treatments have a similar pattern, with a radical inguinal orchidectomy performed first.

- **Seminoma** – Following surgical removal, most men will simply be monitored. For those in whom there is suspicion or indeed evidence of further involvement – for example, lymph node involvement – combination chemotherapy in the form of bleomycin, etoposide and cisplatin (BEP) or etoposide with cisplatin (EP) will often be administered.
- **Nonseminomas** – Treatment will be influenced by the levels of serum tumour markers. Often, for early stage with low tumour marker levels, postsurgery will be actively monitored with regular serum tumour marker checks and CT scans to assess for any signs of spread. With later stage disease or disease that has suspicion of spread, a combination chemotherapy in the form of BEP or EP will be given.
- **Non-GCTs** – Surgery is usually the only treatment required for most Leydig and Sertoli cell tumours, followed by monitoring.

Prostate Gland

The prostate is an accessory gland of the reproductive system and consists of both glandular and muscular tissue. The prostate lies immediately below the bladder, anterior to the rectum and posterior to the pubic ramus. It is about the size of a walnut and is fully mature by the time a man reaches 30; the size remains stable until about the age of 45, when it commonly begins to enlarge (a condition called benign hypertrophy). The prostate is traversed by the urethra, which is lined with transitional cells, and by ejaculatory ducts from the seminal vesicles that join the vas deferens just before entering the prostate. The prostate is an encapsulated, glandular organ with numerous partitions, divided into three zones: peripheral, central and transitional (Fig. 9.3). The peripheral zone is the largest, making up around 70% of the prostate glandular tissue. Moving inwards, the central zone makes up around 25% of the glandular tissue and includes the ejaculatory ducts that ultimately join with the prostatic urethra. Lastly, the transitional zone makes up around 5% of the glandular tissue and contains

a portion of the prostatic urethra. This zone gets its name from the transitional epithelium that sits within. The transitional zone is the area most likely to enlarge and give rise to benign hyperplasia.

Microscopically (Fig. 9.4), each of the glands that constitutes the prostate is surrounded by a basement membrane, which comprises mainly of collagen fibres and basal cells. Interspersed within this basal layer are neuroendocrine cells, specialised cells whose role is not clearly understood but are responsible for various secretions, such as serotonin, calcitonin, chromogranin A and vascular endothelial growth factor (VEGF). Small cell cancer of the prostate is a rare pathology that derives from these neuroendocrine cells. The cells that surround the lumen of the gland are luminal cells, columnar epithelial cells responsible for secreting substances into the prostatic fluid that provide nutrients for the sperm; this forms the bulk of seminal fluid and is a milky fluid of pH 7.4. This is slightly alkaline, which is important as it protects the sperm from the acidic environment present in the male urethra and female vagina. These epithelial cells are also responsible for secreting prostate-specific antigen (PSA), which liquifies semen to allow the sperm to swim freely. Normally, only a small amount of PSA is present in the bloodstream (referred to as serum PSA). High levels of PSA in the blood may indicate overactive epithelial cells within the prostate and are often used to aid the diagnosis of prostate cancer (see later).

ONCOLOGY

Worldwide, cancer of the prostate is one of the most common types of cancer in males. It is the most common form of male cancer in places such as the United Kingdom and United States. The disease is rare before 40, with most men being diagnosed around the age of 75 to 80 years. Generally, it is a slow-growing disease, and many men will live with their prostate cancer and not die from it. Over the last 20 to 30 years, the number of men with prostate cancer has increased. This may be due in part to more men living to ages when it is most common but also because the PSA test has had a very real impact on the number of men diagnosed. The role of the PSA test in diagnosis will be covered later in this chapter.

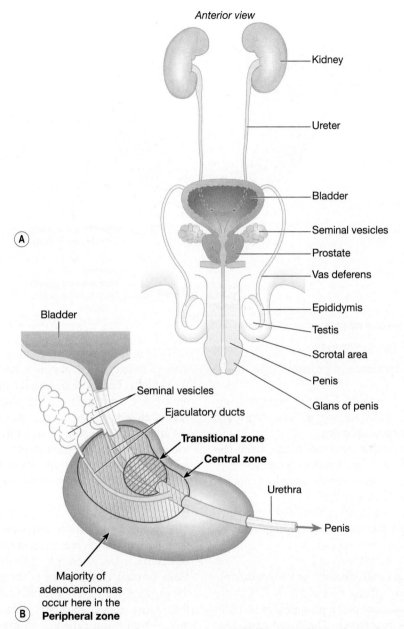

Fig. 9.3 Anatomy of the prostate gland: (A) Relation to other organs *(anterior view)*; (B) 3D cross section showing zonal arrangement.

AETIOLOGY

The underlying aetiologic factors for prostate cancer are not very well known, but there are associated risk factors:

- Age

- Genetic links showing increasing risk with family history; may be associated with mutations in BRCA1 and BRCA2 genes.
- Race-related factors – incidence is lower in Whites than in Blacks. African Americans have

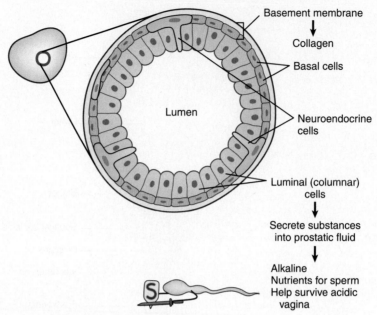

Fig. 9.4 Microscopic view of an individual prostate gland (diagrammatic).

the highest incidence of prostate cancer in the world.

- Geographical variation between countries suggests genetic links are rare in Asia, Africa and South and Central America.
- Diet – higher incidence if diet is rich in fat, particularly red meat; low if rich in vitamin A
- Environment – heavy metals, cadmium, nuclear industry, chemical fertilisers
- Occult cancer – around 15% are discovered incidentally at prostatectomy for benign disease.

HISTOLOGY

The majority of prostate tumours are adenocarcinomas (95%). The peripheral zone (70% to 75% of the gland) is the largest zone of the prostate and accounts for 70% of prostate cancers. The transitional zone (5% of the gland) is the location where benign nodular hyperplasia develops, 20% of which may become adenocarcinoma and may also give rise to transitional cell carcinoma (TCC). The central zone (20% to 25% of the gland) accounts for about 10% of prostate cancers. Small cell cancers arising from the neuroendocrine cells tend to be poorly differentiated, aggressive and early to metastasise. Often, the adenocarcinomas

are well differentiated, although there can be variation throughout. There can be a wide range of tumour differentiation and abnormal histological growth, and this is closely related to the likelihood of metastases and death. Because of this variability within the tumour, many pathologists report the range of differentiation present in the specimen using the Gleason grading scale, discussed in more detail later.

Clinical Features

The symptoms of cancer are often indistinguishable from normal benign enlargement of the prostate. This is a common occurrence in men over the age of 50. Many prostate cancers start in the peripheral zone of the prostate that lies far away from structures, such as the urethra, and, as such, symptoms may not be obvious. Symptomatic patients will experience increased difficulty in micturition (urination), loss of stream strength, hesitancy, postmicturition dribble and the need to urinate frequently (frequency), especially at night (nocturia). About a third of patients present with local invasion and a range of symptoms that include haematuria, tenesmus, impotence, incontinence, loin pain, anuria (inability to urinate) and lymphoedema from acute urinary retention. Some patients will present with metastatic spread, often with bone pain, pathological fracture or sacral, sciatic or perineal pain due to infiltration of nerves in the pelvis.

Direct spread of prostate cancer tends to be to adjacent organs: the bladder, seminal vesicles and rectum. Lymphatic spread is via true pelvic nodes below the bifurcation of the common iliac arteries. Blood-borne spread is common as there is a rich venous plexus lying in front of the vertebral bodies, which may account for a tendency to spread to vertebrae and pelvic bones.

Diagnostic Procedures

There is no general population-based screening test for prostate cancer. However, men of a certain age who are experiencing symptoms may undergo some or all of the following investigations.

Digital Rectal Examination

Digital rectal examination (DRE) can detect abnormalities – the gland feels irregular and hard. It is an inexpensive, quick and easy test. However, it can only detect abnormality in the posterior aspect of the prostate. Also, it cannot really distinguish between benign or malignant disease. Confirmation of malignancy will require further investigations.

Prostate-Specific Antigen Test

PSA is released by the prostate epithelium. It is an indicator of prostate activity, not of prostate cancer. PSA liquifies semen to allow the sperm to swim easily, but only a small amount will be detectable in the circulating blood stream; this is called serum PSA. However, raised levels of serum PSA might indicate malignant disease, but it can be affected by other things, such as certain medical procedures, infection and benign enlargement. Generally, the higher the level of PSA, the more likely a prostate pathology is present. High levels of PSA along with symptoms may indicate the need for further investigations.

Biopsy

The aim here is to take a representative sample of cells around the volume of the prostate. Transrectal ultrasound (TRUS) can be used to image the prostate whilst biopsies are taken. Some centres may use MRI to guide the biopsy or, indeed, transperineal biopsies might be taken under local or general anaesthetic.

Generally, between 12 and 25 core biopsies can be taken. Examination of these biopsies allows pathologists to determine the grade of the tumour and help direct treatment strategy.

Other tests might include blood tests to assess the levels of alkaline phosphatase, as high levels might indicate bone metastases. Symptoms of bone pain and raised alkaline phosphatase may suggest the need for isotope bone scans.

Staging and Grading

Prostate cancer staging uses the TNM system. If clinically detectable disease is present, the important distinction is whether or not the tumour is confined to the prostate. Extension beyond the capsule or, indeed, involvement of other structures, such as the bladder, rectum or seminal vesicles, indicates a worse T classification.

An accurate grade of the prostate cancer is crucial and will help determine the treatment strategy used. The Gleason grading scale provides a measure of the level of differentiation across the tumour and is important as an indicator of how slowly or quickly the disease may progress. The higher the Gleason score, the more likelihood of extracapsular spread, nodal involvement and metastatic disease.

Fig. 9.5 shows a diagrammatic representation of malignant prostate cells from well differentiated (normal looking) to poorly differentiated (very abnormal), with various patterns of differentiation in between.

Each pattern, when seen under a microscope, is given a score between 1 and 5, as seen in the diagram. As described earlier, several biopsies will be taken. Generally, scores of 1 and 2 are ignored as they represent very normal looking cells, whilst scores of 3 or more will be recorded. When looking across the range of biopsies, the pathologist will identify the most common pattern. This is given the initial score. With 'Pattern 1', for example, a score of 3 might be given, indicating moderately differentiated cells. Then the pathologist will look for the worst pattern of the remaining cells within the biopsies. With 'Pattern 2', for example, a score of 4 is given, demonstrating more poorly differentiated cells. Both 'Patterns' are then added together to give the Gleason score, which in this case will be 7 and is written as 7 (3+4). An important note here is that the numbers within the

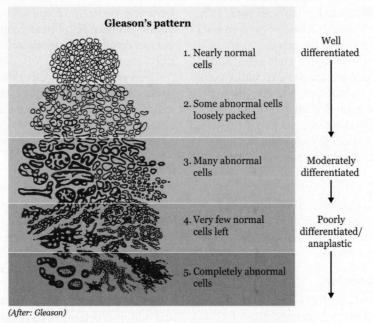

Gleason's pattern

1. Nearly normal cells — Well differentiated

2. Some abnormal cells loosely packed

3. Many abnormal cells — Moderately differentiated

4. Very few normal cells left — Poorly differentiated/ anaplastic

5. Completely abnormal cells

(After: Gleason)

Fig. 9.5 A diagrammatic representation of malignant prostate cancer cells and the level of differentiation.

brackets indicate the score given to the patterns, and their orientation within the brackets is important. In this case, 3 indicates the most common cellular pattern and 4 indicates the worst pattern of the remaining cells.

Gleason scores generally range from 6 (3+3) to 10 (5+5) and are often arranged to grade groups, as seen in Table 9.2. Grade groups, along with the stage, can be useful in determining treatment options.

Treatment

To determine the most appropriate treatment, stage, Gleason score and pre-treatment PSA level are considered. Other factors that affect treatment decisions are the patient's age, personal preference and health status. The aim of treatment is to control spread and reduce tumour cells and allow the patient to live out his life untroubled by disease.

Prostate cancer is generally a slow-growing disease in an older man who is continuing to age. Any treatment intervention at this stage may cause more problems to the man than the disease is giving. Therefore, many men will fall into the 'active surveillance' category of prostate cancer management. Such active surveillance would mean regular PSA testing, maybe

alongside other clinical tests. The aim is to intervene only if the tumour progresses.

In men with localised prostate cancer, there are two main treatment options: radical prostatectomy or radiation therapy. The normal prostate will tolerate high doses of radiation without prostatic symptoms, making external beam radiotherapy a possible treatment option for localised disease. However, there are critical organs (rectum, bladder, erectile nerve) adjacent to the prostate that are very vulnerable to radiation damage, and this can cause serious problems. Brachytherapy is commonly used as an alternative to external beam radiotherapy treatment. The use of implanted radioactive iodine-125 seeds allows a high dose of radiation to be given to the prostate itself with minimal doses to surrounding normal structures. This technique has demonstrated fewer side effects than surgery and external beam radiotherapy, particularly regarding sexual function.

All of the above treatments may be supplemented with hormonal therapies. The cells of the prostate gland are stimulated by male hormones and androgens, in particular testosterone, which is produced by the testes. Most prostate cancers also rely on these hormones for growth and development. The rationale

TABLE 9.2	Gleason Scores and Grade Groups	
Group	**Gleason Score**	**Description**
1	6 (3+3)	All of the cancer cells found look likely to grow slowly.
2	7 (3+4)	Most of the cancer cells found look likely to grow slowly. Some cancer cells look likely to grow at a moderate rate.
3	7 (4+3)	Most of the cancer cells found look likely to grow at a moderate rate. Some cancer cells look likely to grow slowly.
4	8 (3+5)	Most of the cancer cells found look likely to grow slowly. Some cancer cells look likely to grow quickly.
	8 (4+4)	All of the cancer cells found look likely to grow at a moderate rate.
	8 (5+3)	Most of the cancer cells found look likely to grow quickly. Some cancer cells look likely to grow slowly.
5	9 (4+5)	Most of the cancer cells found look likely to grow at a moderate rate. Some cancer cells are likely to grow quickly.
	9 (5+4)	Most of the cancer cells found look likely to grow quickly. Some cancer cells are likely to grow at a moderate rate.
	10 (5+5)	All of the cancer cells found look likely to grow quickly.

for this treatment is either to stop the production of testosterone in the body or to stop the testosterone interacting and binding to the prostate cancer cells. By doing either, the influence of testosterone on the cancer cells is diminished, if not halted altogether, and in the absence of testosterone stimulation, the prostate cancer cells will die.

The production of testosterone by the testes is influenced by hormones, such as LH, secreted by the anterior pituitary gland. This production in the pituitary is influenced by luteinising hormone-releasing hormone (LHRH) by the hypothalamus. LHRH agonist drugs, such as goserelin (Zoladex), leuprorelin (Prostap) and triptorelin (Decapeptyl), are often used. Such 'agonist' drugs promote a rapid release of hormones, especially testosterone, throughout the body before, eventually, the feedback loop to the hypothalamus decreases production of the releasing hormone and, subsequently, levels of testosterone decrease. However, because of the initial surge of testosterone, this can lead to 'tumour flare' in the 2 weeks or so after administration, where the tumour may increase in size and metastases become more painful. Often, it is recommended that anti-androgen therapy be administered at the same time to alleviate some of the results of tumour flare.

Anti-androgen therapies, such as bicalutamide (Casodex), cyproterone acetate (Cyprostat) and flutamide (Drogenil), are a group of drugs that compete for the binding sites for testosterone on the surface of prostate cells and prostate cancer cells, once again limiting the influence of testosterone on these cells. Anti-androgen therapy tends to produce side effects such as:

- Erectile problems (impotence)
- Hot flushes and sweating
- Feeling tired and weak
- Gynaecomastia, breast tenderness

Finally, testosterone levels can be reduced by removing the testicles (orchidectomy; orchiectomy).

Hormone therapies do not get rid of the cancer, and often the prostate cancer will develop resistance to the drugs being used. In this case, chemotherapy in the form of docetaxel (Taxotere) might be used.

The prognosis for prostate cancer is particularly difficult to assess because of the uncertain progress of the disease and the naturally high death rate in this group of elderly men. However, in its earliest stages, many men survive many years with the prostate cancer and die 'with it' rather than 'from it'.

Penis

The penis has two functions: depositing sperm in the female reproductive tract and acting as the terminal duct for the urinary tract to allow the elimination of urine. It consists of an attached root, a free shaft and an enlarged tip.

Internally, the penis is cylindrical; the penile shaft consists of three columns of erectile tissue held together by strong fibrous tissue (Fig. 9.6):

- The corpus cavernosum is made up of two columns forming the major part of the dorsal (uppermost) and lateral (side) volumes of the penis.
- The corpus spongiosum forms the ventral (underside) portion, which expands over the distal end, forming the glans penis, and encases the urethra's proximal end, which is enlarged to form the bulb of the penis.
- The glans penis is a cone-shaped structure formed from corpus spongiosum; its lateral margins form a ridge of tissue known as the corona. The glans is well supplied with sensory receptors.

The male urethra is 20 cm long, commences at the bladder neck and terminates at the urethral orifice on the glans penis. The urethra has three parts:

- The prostatic urethra runs through the prostate and expands into an area called the seminal colliculus into which the seminal vesicle ducts also open.
- The membranous urethra lies between the apex of the prostate and bulb of the penis, surrounded by a sphincter and perineal membrane.
- The spongy urethra passes through the bulb, the corpus spongiosum and the glans penis; immediately before the external urethral orifice, the urethra expands to form the navicular fossa.

The skin of the penis, well supplied with sensory receptors, is a thin, loose skin that covers the penile shaft and includes a fold that extends to cover the glans penis. Called the prepuce (foreskin), this loose fold may be removed by circumcision.

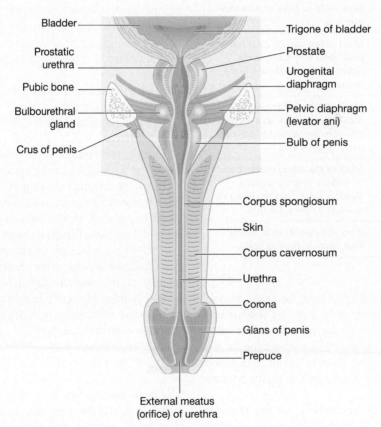

Fig. 9.6 Coronal section view of the penis.

ONCOLOGY

Penile cancer is a rare disease and, when diagnosed early, is very curable. Unfortunately, the outlook worsens with later stage disease. Risk factors include:

- Exposure to the human papilloma virus (HPV), especially HPV16
- Genital warts (mainly due to HPV exposure)
- HIV infection increases risk
- Poor hygiene, smegma, phimosis (inability to retract the foreskin)
- Age; penile cancer is even more rare below 50 years.

Penile carcinomas present almost entirely as squamous cell carcinomas that vary from well to moderately differentiated. Penile carcinomas are usually seen in elderly men who are uncircumcised. The lesion presents as a warty, cauliflower growth that bleeds easily. Penile carcinomas can also present as a solid growth on the shaft, causing ulceration, or may grow insidiously under the foreskin. The lesions are usually slow-growing, and patients often delay diagnosis because of personal embarrassment. Malignant lesions can display a spectrum of changes from dysplasia to carcinoma in situ (also known as erythroplasia of Queyrat or Bowen disease of the penis). These tumours are grouped as penile intraepithelial neoplasia, and many cases are now associated with HPV infection.

Clinically, these symptoms, warty growths on the glans sulcus or base of glans, are often present for over a year before a patient seeks medical help. An infection or bloody discharge can occur under the foreskin. If the lesion is visible, diagnosis is obvious. If phimosis hides it, the glans must be exposed by a dorsal slit in the prepuce or complete circumcision with biopsy. Inguinal nodes may be enlarged, suggesting spread or infection. Blood-borne metastases are rare and late. TNM staging is based around the depth of invasion into the shaft of the penis, with later stages having disease that has penetrated the corpus cavernosum or corpus spongiosum. Invasion of other structures, such as the urethra or prostate, suggest an even worse T classification.

Treatment

Vaccination for HPV, if given to boys, may see a decrease in penile cancer that is HPV related; only time will tell. Generally, treatment is determined by the stage of the disease at presentation.

If the tumour is 'in situ', or superficial, treatment may involve local application of 5-fluorouracil cream or laser therapy. Such procedures may offer a good chance of cure while still preserving cosmetic appearance and sexual function. Once the tumour becomes infiltrative, with or without local skin involvement, the choice of therapy is determined by tumour size, extent of infiltration and the amount of normal tissue destruction. Surgery, partial or total penectomy, is generally the treatment of choice. External beam radiotherapy or brachytherapy might be used if the patient cannot undergo or refuses surgery. If the tumour has metastasised, then chemotherapy might also be an option. Prognosis is very much related to the stage. Men with early-stage disease will do well. Taking into account all stages of the disease, around 50% of men will survive 5 years or more.

SELF-ASSESSMENT QUESTIONS

Answer true or false to the following. Answers are on page 165–166.

1 *The testes are a pair of oval organs that initially develop high up on the anterior wall of the abdomen at about the level of the kidneys.*

2 *The spermatic cord is composed of a muscle, blood, lymph, nerve supply and the vas deferens.*

3 *Each testis contains 200 to 300 compartments called lobules that contain interstitial cells and one to four seminiferous tubules.*

4 *Leydig cells secrete male hormones or androgens, especially testosterone.*

5   *The routes of potential spread of cancer of both the testis and scrotum are the same.*

6   *A history of cryptorchidism is a strong risk factor for developing testicular cancer.*

7   *Testicular cancer is the most common solid tumour in young men aged 15 to 39 years.*

8   *Ninety percent to 95% of testicular tumours are GCTs.*

9   *Treatment management of testicular cancer is based on whether the tumour is of a seminoma or nonseminoma type.*

10   *The prostate is a small organ that lies directly beneath the bladder.*

11   *The prostate gland is divided into three zones: peripheral, transitional and caudal.*

12   *Classically, the symptoms of prostate cancer are very similar to those of benign hyperplasia of the prostate.*

13   *Cancer of the prostate is the most common cancer in males in the United Kingdom.*

14   *Most men are diagnosed with prostate cancer in their 40 s.*

15   *The majority of prostate tumours are adenocarcinomas.*

16   *The peripheral zone is the largest region of the prostate gland and is the zone where the majority of prostatic cancer arises.*

17   *PSA is produced only by the prostate and is a useful tumour marker.*

18   *A patient with prostate cancer with a high Gleason score is likely to experience a long, slow progression and may not develop any symptoms for 10 years or more.*

19   *Penile carcinomas are almost entirely adenocarcinomas.*

20   *Staging is based on the size of the tumour.*

The Female Reproductive System

Objectives

By the end of this chapter, the reader should be able to:

- Outline the anatomy of organs found in the female reproductive system and relate this to the signs and symptoms associated with cancers in these areas.
- Compare and contrast the risk factors associated with cancers found in the female reproductive system.
- Evaluate the role of screening in the diagnosis of cervical and breast cancer.
- Compare and contrast the different types of ovarian cancer and the role of tumour markers in the diagnosis and management of women with ovarian cancer.
- Relate the stages of a breast cancer with possible treatment options.
- Explain the role of HER2, ER and PR in the diagnosis and treatment of breast cancers.
- Understand the role of surgery, radiotherapy, chemotherapy and targeted and hormone therapy in the treatment of female cancers.

The female reproductive system includes the pelvic organs (Fig. 10.1) – comprising the uterus, ovaries, vagina and vulva – along with the breasts, which are classified as external accessory sex organs. The function of the female reproductive system is to produce ova (eggs), provide an environment for a fertilised egg to develop into a foetus and deliver the full-term baby during childbirth. To enable the reproductive organs to fulfil this function, hormones are produced by the ovaries to sustain this cycle of events. The function of the breasts is to provide nutrition for the newborn child in the form of milk; this function is also under the control of hormones.

Point of note: The risk factors for these cancers will be discussed in more detail under each specific

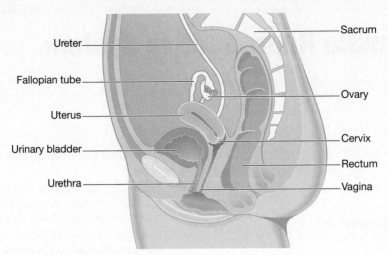

Fig. 10.1 The relational anatomy of the female pelvis.

tumour site, but it is worth noting at this point how similar the risk factors are for cancers of the breast, uterus and ovary. These are very much related to the circulating female hormones, particularly oestrogen. Table 10.1 brings these risk factors together. It can also be noted that the risk factors associated with cervical cancer are very different, mainly related to exposure to the human papilloma virus (HPV), with strains 16 and 18 accounting for around 70% of these cancers.

Uterus

The normal uterus is the size of a medium pear and consists of three parts: the fundus, the body and the cervix. The function of the uterus is to provide an environment for a fertilised egg to develop into a foetus. It is important to note that the cervix is not a separate anatomical organ but is the lower third of the uterus. (The word cervix means neck.) Lying in the pelvic cavity between the bladder in front and the rectum behind (see Fig. 10.1), the size and position of the uterus can vary depending on factors such as age, pregnancy and pelvic organ size. The uterus normally lies flexed over the superior surface of the bladder with the cervix pointing downwards and backwards, joining the vagina at right angles.

The uterine wall has three layers: an outer serous layer (perimetrium), a middle muscular layer (myometrium) and an inner layer (endometrium) (Fig. 10.2).

The perimetrium is the same as the visceral peritoneum in this area, and, the anterior forms the vesicouterine pouch and, posteriorly, the rectouterine pouch. The myometrium has three layers of smooth muscle fibres, which produce coordinated contractions during childbirth to help delivery of the baby. The endometrium has two layers: a permanent layer called the stratum basalis and a surface layer called the stratum functionalis. This inner layer is composed of columnar epithelium, which is in folds, forming numerous glands. The endometrium is under hormonal control and prepares to receive a fertilised egg each month. If fertilisation does not occur, the outer stratum functionalis is removed during menstruation and is replaced by cells from the stratum basalis.

The internal os at the inferior end of the uterus opens out into the cervical canal, which is constricted at its lower end, forming the external os that opens into the vagina (see Fig. 10.2). The cell type changes in this area from columnar to squamous epithelium that is known as the squamous-columnar (or squamocolumnar) junction or transitional zone. This is an area that is tested during cervical screening.

ONCOLOGY

Two different histological types of tumours occur in the uterus, distinguished not only by the different types of tissue but also by very different (and often juxtaposed) causative factors associated with the presenting

TABLE 10.1	Risk Factors Associated With Female Cancers		
Cervix	**Corpus Uterus**	**Ovary**	**Breast**
Risk Factors			
• Human papilloma virus (HPV) (16 & 18) • Smoking • *Safe sex gives protection* • *Vaccine gives protection*	• Early menarche • ↓ Parity • Late menopause • Obesity • Hereditary nonpolyposis colon cancer (gene) Lynch syndrome • Tamoxifen (low)	• No children • Early menarche, late menopause • 5% Hereditary – (sister x3 risk, daughter x6 risk), BRCA1, Lynch syndrome • HRT (oestrogen based) • Obesity • *Contraceptive pill may give protection*	• Early menarche • Late first pregnancy • ↓ Parity • Late menopause • Obesity (post-menopause) • Oral contraceptives and HRT (slight) • Alcohol • 5% Hereditary • Breast density

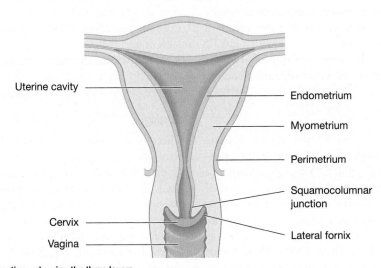

Fig. 10.2 The uterus in sections, showing the three layers.

diseases. The two pathologies are those affecting the body of the uterus and those affecting the cervix.

CARCINOMA OF THE CERVIX

Carcinoma of the cervix is the fourth most common malignancy in women worldwide and is more common in low- to middle-income countries. It is mainly a disease of women in their 40s and 50s, but there is a trend towards higher rates of diagnosis in younger women, which in part can be explained through access to cervical screening, where most screening will start around 25 years of age.

Risk Factors

There are a number of risk factors associated with carcinoma of the cervix, the major factor being exposure to HPV, which can be transmitted through skin-to-skin contact, and most infections occur as a result of intimate sexual contact and penetrative sex. Practising safe sex can reduce the risk of exposure and consequently cervical cancer. Many strains of HPV exist, and it is strains 16 and 18 that cause around 70% of all cervical cancers. Cervical screening programmes worldwide have been very influential in picking up in situ lesions and, as a result, the treatment and subsequent outcome for women with cervical neoplasms has improved dramatically. More recently, the advent of the HPV vaccine has demonstrably reduced the impact of HPV on many girls worldwide, with rates of cervical cancer falling in those populations that have received the vaccine. The HPV vaccine is administered to young girls between 9 and 14 years of age, the rationale being to vaccinate prior to any possible exposure to the virus. A point of note: HPV exposure is linked to other cancers, such as oropharyngeal and anal cancer, and it is hoped that the vaccination programme will lead to further reductions in these types of cancer also. Many countries now also include boys in the vaccination schedule.

Other risk factors include smoking and a reduced immunity. Many of the chemicals found in tobacco smoke have been found in the vaginal mucus, which may explain why cervical cancer is more common in women who smoke. Those women with reduced immunity – for example, those with untreated HIV – are also more prone to the effects of HPV and therefore cervical cancer.

General Pathology

Macroscopically, carcinoma of the cervix appears as a proliferative growth or as an ulcer in the cervical region. The majority (90%) are of squamous cell carcinoma (SCC) type with a few adenocarcinomas. If the tumour is confined to the surface epithelium, it is described as noninvasive. This noninvasive (sometimes referred to as pre-invasive) stage is described as cervical intraepithelial neoplasia (CIN). CIN is graded according to the degree of differentiation, the appearance of the cell nucleus and the mitotic activity and has three levels: CIN I, II and III. CIN III is sometimes referred to as severe dysplasia or carcinoma in situ. A proportion of CIN (particularly CIN III) will eventually progress and become invasive.

Invasive carcinoma, if untreated, will spread in all directions: to the adjoining tissue and organs of the pelvis, including the vaginal vault, the fornices and the endometrium, as well as laterally to the parametria, anteriorly to the bladder, and posteriorly to the rectum. Lymphatic spread can occur to the lymph nodes within the pelvic region, and blood-borne metastases can occur, primarily to the lungs, liver and bone.

Clinical Features

Cervical cancer is often asymptomatic, particularly at an early (CIN) stage, and is often diagnosed from routine cervical screening. Symptoms can include vaginal bleeding, particularly after intercourse, and vaginal discharge. These symptoms are not always picked up quickly as irregular bleeding can be mistaken for menopausal symptoms by women in their 40s and 50s and not reported to the doctor.

Investigations

Further investigation may follow a positive cervical screen. Colposcopy will allow for more detailed examination of the cervix, and this might be followed by removal of the affected area by large loop excision of the transitional zone (LLETZ) or cone biopsy. (LLETZ may also be referred to as LEEP: loop electrosurgical excision procedure.) Both will allow a more detailed look at the cells, assist with staging and grading and inform further treatment, if required. Routine blood tests and CT scans may also be performed, particularly if there is suspicion of wider disease.

Staging

There is a crossover between the TNM staging system and the FIGO (International Federation of Gynaecology and Obstetrics): Both are determined by the level of invasion of any neoplasm and whether the neoplasm is confined to the cervix anatomical area. Early stage would suggest the neoplasm is confined to the cervix only, with later stage indicating involvement of other areas, possibly even other organs, like the urinary bladder. Involvement of lymph nodes and/or evidence of further spread to different parts of the body will indicate stage III and stage IV, respectively.

Treatment

Treatment is largely dictated by stage at presentation. Pre-invasive carcinoma, such as CIN III, will often involve LLETZ or cone biopsy. All have excellent treatment outcomes of nearly 100% and, particularly with LLETZ, will leave the cervix competent. This is important in young women who wish to have children at a future date.

For early-stage invasive carcinoma, surgery and radiotherapy, alone or in combination, are curative.

Factors influencing the choice of treatment include age, the general condition of the patient and the stage of the disease, along with the patient's own preference. Patients may have chemotherapy combined with these modalities to treat obvious or potential systematic disease.

If the tumour is small and confined to the cervix and the patient would still like to bear children, then a trachelectomy may be performed, which removes the cervix and the upper part of the vagina only. More extensive disease will require a hysterectomy, with or without removal of the ovaries. Radiotherapy may be used after surgery for disease which is locally advanced. Normally, it would utilise a combination of internal (brachytherapy) and external irradiation. Chemotherapy, in the form of cisplatin, may be used alongside the radiotherapy (chemoradiation).

Prognosis

Pre-invasive disease like CIN is almost always curable, with treatments like LLETZ being very successful, highlighting the importance of screening and early diagnosis. The outcome for invasive cancers of the cervix is closely related to the stage at presentation, with 5-year survival for early stage being around 95%, but this falls to around 40% and 15% for stages III and IV, respectively.

CANCER OF THE BODY OF THE UTERUS (CORPUS UTERI)

Cancer of the body of the uterus is normally referred to as endometrial carcinoma because it affects the inner lining of the body of the uterus, the endometrium. Tumours arise mainly from the glandular epithelium (adenocarcinomas) and are therefore different in origin from those arising at the cervix. Endometrial carcinoma accounts for approximately 4% of all cancers in women and is mainly a disease of post-menopausal women. Occasionally, sarcomas arise in the muscle leiomyosarcoma.

Risk Factors

The predominant risk factor for endometrial carcinoma is related to exposure to female hormones, particularly oestrogen, over a woman's lifetime (see Table 10.1). Risk factors such as early menarche, late menopause and nulliparous are all related to constant exposure to hormones from an uninterrupted menstrual cycle. Constant exposure to oestrogen and progesterone throughout the menstrual cycle causes constant remodelling of the endometrium, thereby increasing the risk of DNA errors becoming manifest. Obesity, particularly post-menopausal, increases risk also, with fatty deposits able to convert androgens into oestrogen using the catalyst aromatase, furthering the exposure to oestrogen in the post-menopausal setting and endometrial proliferation. Having taken tamoxifen for a previous breast cancer can also increase the risk, although, in the breast, tamoxifen acts more like an oestrogen blocker; it acts more to encourage the proliferation of the endometrial cells in the uterus. A small but significant percentage of cases, around 5%, can be attributed to hereditary syndromes such as Lynch syndrome. If such cases are identified, then others within that family unit may be screened and counselled.

Pathology

Macroscopically, tumours arising within the uterine cavity may be polypoid or diffuse multifocal growths. They arise from the glandular epithelium of the endometrium, and microscopically they are predominantly adenocarcinomas, the majority being well differentiated. Sarcomas may arise from the muscular layer of the uterus but are rare.

It may be that endometrial cancer is categorised according to its propensity to be aggressive and spread. Type 1 cancers are the most common and are very much associated with excess oestrogen in the body. Type 2 is less common but tends to be more aggressive. It is not hormone dependent and will include serous and clear cell carcinomas.

Clinical Features

The classic presentation of endometrial carcinoma is irregular bleeding, in particular, post-menopausal bleeding. As in cervical carcinoma, this may not be reported early as it may be thought of as a normal menopausal symptom. Endometrial carcinoma may also be detected as an incidental finding during cervical screening. Investigations would include histological diagnosis by hysteroscopy and biopsy. A chest x-ray may be done to exclude metastases, along with a CT scan to assess local spread and lymph node status.

Staging

Once again, there is crossover here between the TNM and FIGO staging systems. Generally, the stage will be dependent on whether the cancer is confined to the uterus, invaded into the myometrium and/or involves other areas. Lymphatic spread to the regional lymph nodes of the pelvic cavity and para-aortic lymph nodes will be assessed, and there is possibility of late spread via the blood to the lungs and bones.

Treatment

Surgery is the main form of treatment for endometrial carcinoma and generally takes the form of a total hysterectomy, possibly with removal of the ovaries (bilateral salpingo-oophorectomy).

Radiotherapy may be used postoperatively and can be given as external beam, brachytherapy or a combination of both. Chemotherapy (cisplatin and paclitaxel) may be given if advanced disease or for type 2 cancers. For patients with late-stage disease who may not be well enough for surgery, some response and relief of symptoms can be gained with the administration of progesterone, with drugs such as medroxyprogesterone acetate (Provera) and megestrol (Megace).

Prognosis

The prognosis overall is good, as the majority of patients present with stage I disease. Around 90% 5-year survival for stage I disease can be achieved. For advanced disease, 5-year survival rates fall to 65% for stage II and 20% for stage IV.

Ovary

Each ovary (Fig. 10.3) is the size and shape of a large almond. The ovaries are located below and behind the uterine tubes at the side of the uterus and are attached to the uterus by a ligament. The end of the uterine (fallopian) tube curves over the ovary but is not attached to it. The ovary has two functions: ovulation and hormone secretion. The ovary is covered by a layer of germinal epithelium, although this is perhaps misleading as it is not the tissue that develops the ova. The ova are found in structures called ovarian follicles that are embedded in connective tissue toward the centre of the ovary. These follicles consist of an oocyte surrounded by specialised hormone-secreting cells (granulosa). The oocytes are under the influence of follicle-stimulating hormone (FSH), which is produced by the pituitary gland. The oocytes start to grow each month following puberty. FSH also stimulates the secretion of oestrogen by the follicles. Other hormones then become involved to stimulate ovulation and further production of oestrogen along with progesterone. This monthly menstrual cycle is in three phases. In the first or menstrual phase, the inner lining of the endometrium is lost; during this phase the ovarian follicles also begin their development. The second phase or pre-ovulatory stage is when the follicles produce oestrogen to stimulate the repair of the endometrium and the follicle becomes ready for ovulation. Ovulation occurs when an immature ovum is released into the pelvic cavity. The final stage is the post-ovulatory stage, when the endometrium starts to thicken in preparation for fertilisation and implantation of the embryo. If this does not occur, the cycle repeats itself and menstruation and follicular development start again.

ONCOLOGY

Ovarian cancer is a disease that kills more women than any other gynaecologic malignancy. Even with aggressive treatment, the survival rates are poor. Early detection would save lives, but the manifestation of the disease makes this problematic, with often vague or no symptoms at the start. There are around 7500 new cases of ovarian cancer in the United Kingdom each year, with over 4000 deaths per year. There is a similar incidence in the United States, accounting for around 21,000 cases and 14,000 deaths per year.

Risk Factors

Ovarian carcinoma tends to occur in women over 40 years, with a peak age of incidence between 70 and 79 years. Known risk factors seem to be associated with continued ovulation throughout a woman's lifetime. Early menarche and late menopause are therefore associated risk factors. Constant ovulation produces constant pitting and repair of the surface of the ovary. It is thought that this constant process of repairing damaged parts of the ovary increases the risk of epithelial ovarian cancers. Because of this, women who have no children tend to be at higher risk. During pregnancy, the body ceases to produce ova and therefore ovulation, reducing the exposure to the constant repair mechanism. Certain ovarian cancers are related

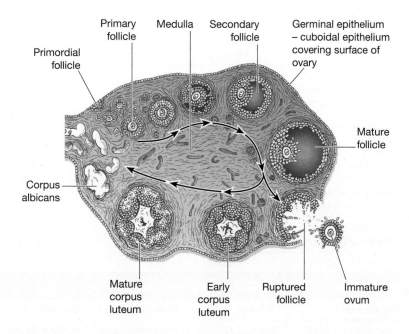

Fig. 10.3 The ovary in section, showing the developmental stages of the ovarian cycle.

to genetic factors (around 5%). Mutated BRCA 1 and 2 increases risk, as does Lynch syndrome.

Interestingly, the incidence of ovarian cancer has declined somewhat over the last 10 to 20 years. It is thought that this is a benefit of taking oral contraceptives that prevent ovulation and thus the pitting and repair mechanism described earlier. The longer the contraceptive pill is taken, the greater the protection against ovarian cancer. Another point of note: Use of oral contraceptives will increase, if only slightly, the risk of breast and uterine cancer.

Pathology

There is a wide variety of tumour cell types, 90% of which arise from the surface epithelium. Of these, 10% are borderline malignancy with no invasion; 1% to 2% arise from germ cells, which are more common in young women; and 2% arise from specialised hormone-producing cells (see Tables 10.2–10.4). Secondary tumours can also occur in the ovary from carcinoma of the uterus, breast or gastrointestinal tract (Krukenberg tumours).

EPITHELIAL TUMOURS

The tumours arise from the surface epithelium of the ovary. Serous carcinoma is the most common (see Table 10.2). CA125 is a tumour marker that can be secreted by serous and mucinous types but is used more as a monitor to assess effectiveness of treatment rather than as a screening tool. Rarely, a patient may present with widespread deposits of tumour throughout the peritoneum. Such primary peritoneal cancers are generally serous carcinomas indistinguishable from serous epithelial carcinoma of ovary and arise from cells lining the peritoneum and will be treated in same way as other ovarian epithelial cancers.

GERM CELL TUMOURS

Germ cell tumours derive from the cells which will ultimately become the ova, and their characteristics are listed in Table 10.3. Dysgerminoma is the most common type and is very similar to seminoma of the testes. Elevation of hCG and LDH may aid in diagnosis and management. Yolk sac tumours predominantly affect young women and girls. These rapid-growing

TABLE 10.2 Ovarian Epithelial Tumour Characteristics

	Serous	Mucinous	Brenner	Endometroid
Who	Post-menopausal BRCA1, Lynch syndrome Multiparity is protective			
Histology	Gland-like structures with clear fluid Thought to arise from fallopian tube Associated on pathology with psammoma bodies (round calcium deposits)	Gland-like structures with mucus	Cysts, lined with transitional epithelium Transitional cell carcinoma	Endometrial, gland-like tissue, often associated with other lesions in uterus and endometriosis Often low grade
Tumour markers	CA 125 – not diagnostic but to assess tumour burden after treatment			

TABLE 10.3 Characteristics of Ovarian Germ Cell Tumours

	Dysgerminoma	Yolk Sac	Chorio-Carcinoma	Teratoma
Who	Most common type Pre-menopausal	Pre-menopausal Often children	Pre-menopausal	Younger women
Histology	Fried egg appearance Large cells, clear cytoplasm, large nuclei	Schiller Duvel bodies	Placental-like tissue	Mixed cell types Mature (benign) most common or immature (malignant)
Gross appearance			Very small tumours; early to mets.	Mature tissue, including hair, teeth, skin etc. Can be bilateral
Markers	PLAP, β-hCG, LDH	Alpha-fetoprotein (AFP)	hCG	

β-hCG, Beta-human chorionic gonadotrophin; LDH, lactate dehydrogenase; PLAP, placental-like alkaline phosphatase.

TABLE 10.4 Characteristics of Ovarian Sex Cord Stromal Tumours

	Granulosa Cell	Sertoli-Leydig Cell (Androblastoma)
Who	Mostly per-imenopausal Most common type	Mostly pre-menopausal (< 30 years)
Histology	Call Exner bodies	Reinke crystals (hollow or solid tubes surrounded by Sertoli cells Mostly benign
Gross appearance	Yellow appearance due to presence of lipids in cells	
Markers	Oestrogen, inhibin	Androgen
Physiology	Signs of excess oestrogen; e.g., post-menopausal bleeding, precocious puberty	Signs of excess androgen; e.g., virilisation – hair growth, voice deepening

tumours, often with early lymphatic spread, often have raised AFP, which again can be used to aid diagnosis and monitor response to therapy. Choriocarcinoma derives from placental-like tissue and, as such, will often display high levels of beta-hCG. This tumour is often early to metastasis but is very responsive to chemotherapy treatment. Teratomas are more often benign or benign-like in the ovary compared to the testes, where they behave with more malignant potential. Teratomas in the ovary often contain deposits of fully mature tissue, with such things as hair, skin, teeth and even eyes being found in histological specimens.

SEX CORD STROMAL TUMOURS

These rare tumours are thought to arise from the stromal component of the developing gonad. Granulosa cells surround the developing ovum and secrete oestrogen and inhibin. Elevated levels of these with associated physical manifestations will aid in diagnosis. Sertoli-Leydig tumours, also known as androblastomas, are a rare tumour that often secretes androgens with associated signs (see Table 10.4).

Clinical Features

Ovarian tumours tend to grow slowly and silently for a long time and, as a result, they are usually at an advanced stage at diagnosis. Sixty percent will have spread outside the pelvis at presentation, and some tumours, particularly benign tumours, can attain sizes resembling an advanced pregnancy and eventually cause pressure symptoms. In hormone-producing tumours, the first symptoms may be from the action of the hormones, rather than from the growth itself.

Lymphatic spread to the para-aortic nodes and blood-borne metastases to liver and lungs occur late. Most tumours are cystic and spread to the outer peritoneal surface or the cyst ruptures into the peritoneal cavity. Cells become attached to or invade adjacent structures, including the fallopian tubes, uterus, large and small bowel and bladder. Deposits from ruptured tumours may seed through the peritoneal cavity to other peritoneal surfaces as high up as the diaphragm.

Investigations

Routine tests are often unremarkable, although in advanced cases there may be electrolyte disturbance from intestinal obstruction or ureteric obstruction causing renal failure. A laparotomy is necessary to assess the extent of the disease. Ultrasound of ovaries and liver, along with CT scan of abdomen and pelvis, can demonstrate primary tumour, lymph nodes and liver metastases, if present.

There are various tumour markers that can help in the diagnosis of ovarian cancer and also aid in monitoring the effectiveness of treatment (see Tables 10.2–10.4). CA125 has long been investigated as a possible screening tool, but it can be raised for other reasons and indeed normal for some women with ovarian cancer. This lack of sensitivity and specificity means it is not reliable enough, at least as yet, to be used as a national screening programme.

Staging

Staging for ovarian cancer utilises the TNM and FIGO systems, and important factors include whether the tumour is confined to the ovary and if there is evidence of peritoneal spread (malignant ascites).

Treatment

The primary treatment for ovarian carcinoma is surgery. All patients with operable disease should have a laparotomy and total abdominal hysterectomy with bilateral salpingo-oophorectomy. Both ovaries are removed, as a significant number of tumours are bilateral or carry the risk of metastatic disease to the contralateral ovary. It may be possible to remove only the affected ovary in young women, as long as the tumour is confirmed to be unilateral, well differentiated and mucinous and the peritoneum is found to be negative. Following surgery, other forms of treatment may be given, depending on the stage of the disease. Stage I disease with normal postoperative CT scan and normal CA125 levels requires no further treatment other than close observation. Patients with stage II and III disease should have chemotherapy, usually a combination of cisplatin and paclitaxel. Stage IV disease with soft tissue metastases has a poor prognosis.

PARP (poly (ADP-ribose) polymerase) inhibitor drugs may be used for advanced ovarian cancer that is deemed BRCA related. Both PARP and BRCA are a family of proteins that are involved in several cellular processes, involving mainly DNA repair and programmed cell death. PARP repairs single-strand breaks in DNA, and if left unrepaired, this will become a double-strand break. BRCA is responsible for repairing double-strand breaks. PARP and BRCA work together to form an effective DNA repair mechanism for cells (Fig. 10.4). Cancer that contains mutated BRCA effectively means that the double-strand damage repair mechanism is not working. Using PARP inhibitor drugs like olaparib (Lynparza) can shut down the second repair mechanism, making damage caused by DNA-damaging chemotherapy more effective.

Prognosis

Early-stage disease offers good survival, with 95% of those with stage I surviving more than 5 years. Unfortunately, more than half of patients will present with late-stage disease; less than 40% of those with stage III disease survive more than 5 years, and this drops to less than 20% for stage IV.

Vagina and Vulva

VAGINAL CANCER

Primary tumours of the vagina are rare, accounting for around 750 cases per year in the United Kingdom. Most occur in patients aged 75 years or over in the upper vagina; approximately 90% are SCC, and 10% are adenocarcinomas. The main risk factor is HPV (16) infection, and it may be difficult to differentiate between a vaginal or cervical primary in some cases, and biopsy will be required to confirm diagnosis. Vaginal bleeding tends to be the most common symptom.

Staging is based on whether the disease is confined to the vaginal canal or has extended into the muscle or other pelvic areas. The most common treatment is surgery. For those who cannot have surgery, or if there is post-surgery residual tumour, then radiotherapy with either interstitial or intracavitary radiotherapy can be used. Prognosis is very much related to stage, with 75% 5-year survival at stage I to 20% for stage IV.

VULVAR CANCER

Vulvar cancer is rare, predominantly affecting elderly women. There is an association with viral infections such as HPV. Tumours are exophytic or ulcerative and may have an associated leucoplakia. Virtually all are SCCs and may be preceded by vulva intraepithelial neoplasia (VIN). Symptoms include vulvar itching (70%), discharge and bleeding.

Surgery is the treatment of choice, along with regional node dissection to prevent unsalvageable recurrence. Radiotherapy may be used postoperatively both locally and to the lymphatics. Prognosis is good if lymphatics are not involved, with a 5-year survival of up to 80%, but this drops to below 50% in cases with lymphatic involvement.

Breast

The breasts, which are external accessory sex organs, lie on the anterior chest wall, attached to the pectoral muscles by a layer of connective tissue. Adult female breasts are composed of glandular, adipose (fatty) and fibrous tissue (Fig. 10.5). Glandular tissue comprises

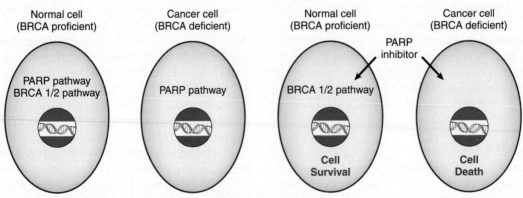

Fig. 10.4 Role of poly (ADP-ribose) polymerase inhibitors in BRCA mutated cancer.

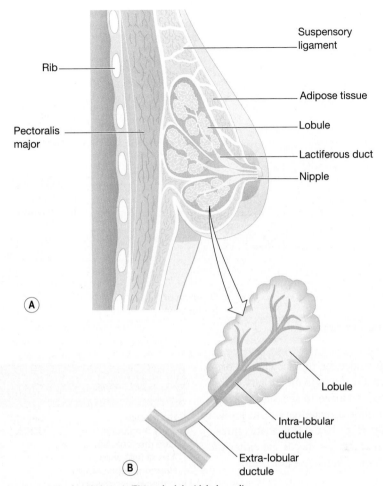

Rib

Pectoralis major

Suspensory ligament

Adipose tissue

Lobule

Lactiferous duct

Nipple

(A)

Lobule

Intra-lobular ductule

Extra-lobular ductule

(B)

Fig. 10.5 (A) Sagittal section through the female breast; (B) terminal duct lobular unit.

15 to 20 lobes in each breast, which are further divided into lobules composed of secretory alveoli arranged around small ducts or ductules (see Fig. 10.5A). These small ductules unite to form one lactiferous duct for each lobe and converge at the nipple, opening at individual orifices on the surface of the nipple. Fibrous tissue known as Cooper ligaments supports the lobules, with adipose tissue lying over the gland and between the lobes. The size of the breast is related to the amount of adipose tissue, not the amount of glandular tissue, and therefore size does not relate to functional ability.

Until puberty, both males and females have small amounts of breast tissue consisting of a few ducts. Breast development in the female occurs at puberty and is controlled by the female hormones oestrogen and progesterone. Oestrogen is responsible for stimulating duct growth and progesterone for stimulating the development of the alveoli and secreting cells. In males, testosterone production prevents further growth development. The function of the female breast is secretion of milk via the lactiferous ducts and nipple.

From an oncology perspective, the lymphatic drainage of the breast is critically important as spread of the disease and prognosis are directly related to lymphatic involvement. Two sets of lymphatic vessels drain the breast: those that originate in the skin and those that originate in the breast itself, including the nipple. Those in the skin form a cutaneous lymphatic plexus that connects with breast tissue lymphatics via

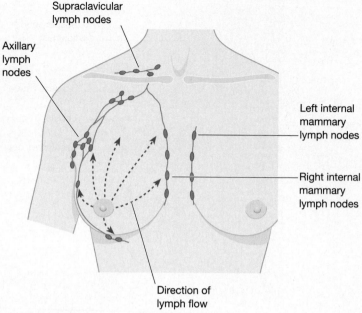

Fig. 10.6 Lymphatic drainage of the right breast.

the subareolar plexus under the nipple. The majority of breast lymph eventually drains to the axillary lymph nodes, with additional drainage to the supraclavicular nodes and to the internal mammary (also known as 'parasternal') nodes (Fig. 10.6). Lymphatic spread from one breast to the other can occur via either the superficial or breast tissue lymphatics but is rare.

ONCOLOGY

Breast cancer is the most common form of malignancy in women in the developed world, and it is estimated that around one in nine women will develop breast cancer at some point in their lives, although it mainly affects women aged 40 to 70 years. Incidence increases with age and is rare below 30 years of age. The incidence of breast cancer is rising, with around 56,000 cases per year in the United Kingdom. Male breast cancer is rare and accounts for only 1% of all breast cancers.

Risk Factors

The risk factors associated with female breast cancer are outlined in Table 10.5.

Genetic predisposition with mutations in the BRCA genes will give rise to around 6% of breast cancers in

TABLE 10.5 **Risk Factors Associated With Female Breast Cancer**	
Hormones	**Genetic**
Early menarche	BRCA 1 and 2
Late menopause	
Age at first child	
Hormone replacement therapy, contraceptive pill	
Lifestyle	**Other**
Diet	Age
Post-menopausal obesity	Dense breast tissue
Alcohol	Benign disease

women. Around 50% to 70% of women with mutated BRCA 1 or 2 will develop breast cancer before 70 years. Women diagnosed with mutated BRCA genes will generally be offered regular screening, usually MRI or ultrasound, so that any cancer can be picked up early. Some may opt for prophylactic double mastectomies to reduce the risk of any breast cancer occurring.

The breast is continuously under hormonal influence, and breast tissue does not fully mature until after the woman has undergone a full-term pregnancy, when the body has undergone its full hormone cycle. There are many factors that link breast cancer with a hormonal cause. There is an increased incidence in women who start menarche early with an associated late menopause and therefore have a longer time when oestrogens are active within the body. Having no children or having them later in life also has been shown to be a risk factor and may be related to the lack or late maturation of the breast tissue. The use of contraceptive pills and hormone replacement therapy can increase the risk of breast cancer if used long term, although it is thought that hormone replacement therapy probably promotes the growth of an existing tumour rather than initiating malignant change. Hormone replacement therapy also has many benefits for women's health, including a protective function against osteoporosis, and it is therefore important that the risks and benefits be discussed on an individual basis.

Diet and obesity are also known risk factors in the development of breast cancer. Pre-menopausal women have a reduced risk if they have a high body mass index or gain weight during adult life, whereas in post-menopausal women there is an increased risk with high body mass index, thought to be related to increased oestrogen production from adipose tissue, and this association is greater with increasing age and years after menopause.

Clinical Features

Breast tumours are often found by the patient or her partner as a painless lump in the breast. Increasingly, smaller tumours are being found through the breast screening programme, although it has not been as successful in detecting early curable disease as the cervical screening programme. At present, the screening programme is primarily for women 50 to 70 years of age, with some regional variations. Greater sensitivity of the screening programme has led to an increase in 'in situ' lesions being detected. Other features of the disease, if not picked up early, are inversion of the nipple, distortion of overlying skin, inflammation of all or part of the breast and fungation, if left very late.

Pathology

Breast disease may be benign, in situ or invasive. Benign disease includes cysts, fibroadenomas and papillomas; lesions arising in the ducts and lobes are referred to as either ductal carcinoma in situ (DCIS) or lobular carcinoma in situ (LCIS). 'In situ' refers to the fact that the malignant cells are confined to the ducts or lobes, and a proportion have the potential to become invasive. Invasive tumours indicate that the malignant cells have broken through the basement membrane and are directly invading the surrounding tissue. They develop mainly from the glandular tissue (ducts and lobes) and are therefore adenocarcinomas.

DCIS was relatively unheard of prior to the advent of breast screening, with most cases being asymptomatic and around 90% detected via mammography. DCIS can be categorised into three grades, low, intermediate and high, based on levels of mitotic activity, necrosis and cellular pleomorphism. In some cases, it may progress to invasive cancer; low-grade DCIS tends to progress to low-grade invasive cancer and high-grade DCIS to high-grade invasive cancers. It is possible that some low-grade DCIS will never progress to an invasive state at all, and this calls into question the role of any treatment intervention in this group. Pure DCIS is not a threat to life, and any treatment intervention is aimed at preventing any possible progression to an invasive state.

Histological grading of invasive breast cancer is important, as it determines the management of the patient and correlates with local recurrence rate as well as the overall prognosis of the disease. Grading is based on three factors, nuclear pleomorphism, mitotic activity and the degree of glandular formation, and three grades, grade 1 (low), grade 2 and grade 3 (high) are indicated. It is imperative that a histological diagnosis be made, as this, along with the TNM staging, is important in management decisions for the patient. As previously mentioned, lymphatic spread is an important aspect of the diagnosis and prognosis of breast cancer. Sampling and histological assessment of the axillary nodes also must be considered when patient management decisions are being made. Sentinel node biopsies will help in determining which lymph nodes are involved. Breast cancer also spreads via the blood to the bones, liver, lungs and brain.

IMPORTANT BIOMARKERS

Two (and maybe three) important biomarkers will be assessed.

HER2 (neu, EbrB2) is a protein receptor found on the surface of cells. It is a growth factor that can be overexpressed on breast cancer cells. Overexpression of *HER2* gene causes cells to over-proliferate. Between 15% and 25% of patients with breast cancer will have this defective gene in their breast cancer cells. Trastuzumab (Herceptin) is a monoclonal antibody that blocks the action of this gene and is an important addition to the treatment for patients with HER2-positive breast cancer. Patients with HER2-positive disease tend to have better survival, probably due to the advent of Herceptin.

Herceptin does have side effects: fatigue, feverish chills, diarrhoea and aches and pains and, importantly, it damages the heart. Therefore, patients with existing heart problems will need to be monitored very carefully.

Oestrogen receptor status is another important biomarker. Breast cells are very responsive to the oestrogen hormone, as are some breast cancer cells. The oestrogen molecule binds to the oestrogen receptor on the cell surface and sets up a signal cascade that results in increased proliferation. Over-expression of the oestrogen receptors on the surface of breast cancer cells means a heightened and increased signal cascade that will promote growth and proliferation. Blocking the receptor with tamoxifen will limit the cell's exposure to oestrogen and dampen down the proliferation signal. Tamoxifen will often be used alongside the other therapies in pre-menopausal women.

In post-menopausal women with breast cancer who are oestrogen positive, a different approach may be required, as excess circulating oestrogens will be depleted. However, oestrogen is still about in the female body, particularly if the women remain obese. Aromatase is a catalyst which coverts androgens into oestrogen in the post-menopausal setting and, as such, aromatase inhibitor drugs, such as anastrozole (Arimidex), letrozole (Femara) or exemestane (Aromasin) may be utilised. Once again, women with oestrogen positive breast cancer generally have a better outcome.

A third marker, progesterone, may be assessed. Although helpful in understanding the development of breast cancer, progesterone receptor targeting is not yet routinely used in the treatment of breast cancer.

Point to note: If a breast cancer is negative for HER2, negative for oestrogen and negative for progesterone, it is said to be *triple negative*. Women with triple negative breast cancer (around 15% of cases) tend to have disease that is more aggressive and more likely to metastasise. Coupling this with the fact that only the standard treatments of surgery, chemotherapy and radiotherapy can be employed means that survival is lower in this group.

Staging

Generally, the TNM staging system is used. The T classification is based on the size of the tumour. T1 suggests it is smaller than 2 cm in its greatest dimension, whereas T3 would indicate a lesion greater than 5 cm. T4 indicates direct extension beyond the breast. The N classification indicates evidence of involvement (or not) of ipsilateral (same side) lymph nodes and will often be a pathological classification indicated by a lowercase 'p' on pathology reports.

Treatment

DCIS is usually treated with mastectomy or wide local excision, which may be followed up by radiotherapy. The aim of this treatment is to prevent any possible progression to an invasive cancer. The debate continues around treatment for those women with low-grade DCIS and whether a 'watch and wait' strategy might suffice.

Women with invasive breast cancer will almost always be offered surgery, either mastectomy or lumpectomy, as the first treatment. After lumpectomy, radiotherapy may be employed to treat the rest of the breast tissue and maybe associated lymphatics. The use of chemotherapy will be influenced by the grade, with patients having high-grade disease being more likely to receive chemotherapy combinations, such as docetaxel, doxorubicin (Adriamycin) and cyclophosphamide (TAC) or cyclophosphamide, methotrexate and fluorouracil (CMF). On occasion, for large tumours, chemotherapy may be given neo-adjuvantly to shrink the tumour prior to surgery.

Those women with HER2-positive breast cancer will benefit from the inclusion of Herceptin in the treatment protocol, and those with oestrogen-positive disease will receive tamoxifen or aromatase inhibitor drugs.

SELF-ASSESSMENT QUESTIONS

Answer true or false to the following. Answers are on page 165–166.

1. *The uterus consists of two parts: the fundus and the body.*

2. *The endometrial lining is under hormonal control.*

3. *The FIGO staging system is often used for gynaecological cancers.*

4. *Cervical cancer is mainly a disease of women over 40 years of age.*

5. *Exposure to the HPV is an important risk factor for carcinoma of the cervix.*

6. *HPV vaccinations give 100% protection against cervical cancer.*

7. *Most cervical cancers are adenocarcinomas.*

8. *Uterine cancer tends to affect younger women.*

9. *Post-menopausal obesity is a known risk factor for uterine cancer.*

10. *The majority of endometrial carcinomas are SCCs.*

11. *Most ovarian cancers are germ cell tumours.*

12. *Ovarian carcinoma occurs more in women with many children.*

13. *Teratoma of the ovary tends to be benign.*

14. *Choriocarcinoma derives from placental-like tissue and as such will often display high levels of β-hCG.*

15. *CA125 is often raised in all types of ovarian cancer.*

16. *Breast size is related to the number of lobules.*

17. *Most breast lymph drains to the axillary nodes.*

18. *Most breast cancers will be classed as HER2+ve.*

19. *DCIS is more common than invasive cancers of the breast.*

20. *ER+ve breast cancer can be treated with Herceptin, alongside other therapies.*

Lung Cancer

Chapter Outline

Objectives

By the end of this chapter, the reader should be able to:

- Describe the relational anatomy of the lungs.
- Outline the main types of cells and tissues found in the lung and relate this to the different types of lung cancer.
- Explain the role of smoking as the major risk factor for lung cancer and its impact on lung cancer incidence and mortality.
- Compare and contrast small cell and non–small cell lung cancer.
- Understand the role of epidermal growth factor receptor (EGFR), *ALK, KRAS* and other genetic mutations found in lung cancer.
- Outline the role of surgery, radiotherapy, chemotherapy and targeted therapy in the treatment of lung cancer.

The trachea or windpipe (Fig. 11.1) is a continuation of the larynx. It is lined with ciliated epithelium and is supported by C-shaped cartilaginous rings joined together posteriorly by the trachealis muscle. The C-shaped supporting structure allows the oesophagus, which is posterior to the trachea, to distend into it when food is swallowed. The function of the trachea is simple but important in that it maintains an open passageway for the flow of air to and from the lungs. The trachea bifurcates at the carina into the right and left main bronchi. Normally, the right bronchus is slightly larger and more vertical than the left. The bronchi resemble the trachea in structure, with incomplete cartilaginous rings. As the bronchi enter the lungs at the hilum, the cartilaginous rings become whole, and the bronchus immediately divides into secondary bronchi. The bronchi continue to divide into smaller and smaller tubes called bronchioles and finally form alveoli, where the exchange of gases occurs. It is difficult to identify when bronchus

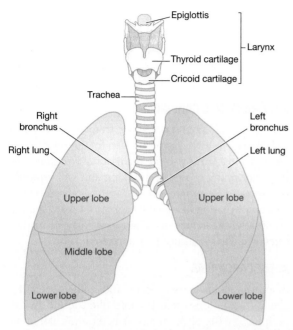

Fig. 11.1 Anatomical relationship of the larynx, trachea, bronchi and lungs.

Labels: Epiglottis, Thyroid cartilage, Cricoid cartilage, Larynx, Trachea, Right bronchus, Right lung, Left bronchus, Left lung, Upper lobe, Upper lobe, Middle lobe, Lower lobe, Lower lobe

becomes lung and therefore carcinomas of the bronchus and lung tend to be grouped together.

The lungs are cone-shaped organs that sit on top of the diaphragm and extend superiorly to a level just above the clavicles. The ribs encase the lungs for protection. Their medial edge is concave, with the left being slightly more concave to allow room for the heart. The main bronchus and pulmonary vessels enter and leave at the hilum of the lung. Each lung is divided into lobes by fissures. The left lung is divided into two lobes, superior (upper) and inferior (lower), and the right lung is divided into three lobes, superior, middle and inferior. The visceral pleura covers the outer surface of the lung.

The lungs are served by a very rich lymphatic drainage network that starts with the internal pulmonary nodes. Drainage then continues to the broncho-pulmonary nodes near the hilum of the lung and onto the trachea-bronchial nodes near the carina area, then to the broncho-mediastinal nodes, and finally to the thoracic duct or right lymphatic duct. A point of note: the superior vena cava, a major vein bringing blood back to the heart from the head and neck, traces its path through the area near to these lymph nodes. In

advanced lung cancer cases, these lymph nodes may enlarge and compress the superior vena cava and restrict the flow of blood. This is referred to as a superior vena caval obstruction or SVCO. Symptoms will include difficulty breathing, puffed-up neck and face, and bulging veins, among others. Palliative radiotherapy to reduce the swollen nodes and allow blood to flow more freely will alleviate symptoms.

Furthermore, the physiology of the lungs is designed to bring oxygenated blood back to the heart and out to the circulation as quickly and efficiently as possible and, as such, has a very rich blood circulation surrounding the very fragile alveoli structures. Lung cancers can easily invade these blood vessels and be taken quickly back to the heart and out to circulation. Such physiology makes for a ready-made 'metastatic highway' for lung cancers, and unfortunately, many patients will present already with metastatic spread, making curative treatments challenging.

Oncology

Around 46,000 new cases of lung cancer present each year in the United Kingdom, making it the second most common form of cancer. It is the most common form of cancer death worldwide, with tobacco use the most common cause. Smoking is directly implicated in 90% of lung cancer cases, and the risk is related to the number of cigarettes smoked and the length of time since the person started smoking. Over the last 30 years, there has been a gradual decrease in male lung cancer, whereas the same time frame has seen a gradual increase in female lung cancer incidence, although this has started to plateau and now decrease. The mid-1970s saw a male-to-female ratio of around 4:1 of lung cancer cases, which is now very close to 1:1. Such changes in incidence reflect smoking habits and smoking cessation trends. Throughout this time period, there was a reduction in the number of men smoking, whilst women as a population started to take up smoking. Such changes in smoking habits are reflected in the changes in lung cancer incidence.

There is an increased risk of lung cancer in partners of people who smoke and those exposed to environmental tobacco smoke (ETS), otherwise known as second-hand smoke, or passive smoke, indicating that passive smoking is an important causative factor.

Tobacco smoke contains many carcinogens (around 70), and the ETS that others inhale is unfiltered, making it a very harmful substance. It is difficult to quantify how much passive smoke a person may inhale, but there remains no known safe limit. Overexposure to passive smoke is thought to increase the risk of lung cancer by around 25%, and 15% of lung cancers may be caused by exposure to passive smoke. Other factors implicated in the presentation of lung cancer are environmental factors, such as air pollution and industrial hazards – for example, exposure to nickel and chrome.

Pathology

Lung cancer is actually two major disease processes identified by cell type: small cell carcinoma (small or oat cell) and 'non–small cell' carcinoma, also referred as non-small cell lung cancer (NSCLC) (everything else). There are four main histologies: small cell (or oat cell) carcinoma, SCC (the most common), large cell carcinoma and adenocarcinoma (Box 11.1). Adenosquamous carcinoma and undifferentiated carcinoma may also be classified as 'non–small cell' carcinoma.

SMALL CELL LUNG CANCER

Small cell lung cancer is often referred to as 'oat' cell as it is composed of primitive-looking cells smaller than normal cells with very large nuclei that resemble oats under a microscope. This cancer is thought to originate from the neuroendocrine cells within the lung that are thought to monitor oxygen levels in the body. Such cells may oversecrete various hormones, typically antidiuretic hormone (ADH) and adrenocorticotrophic hormone (ACTH), leading to various para-neoplastic syndromes, such as Cushing syndrome. This disease is very much related to smoking and will often arise in the main bronchi. It is a very rapidly growing tumour, and many patients will present with metastases, making treatment options limited.

SQUAMOUS CELL CARCINOMA

Squamous cell carcinoma arises from the squamous cells lining the airways and is often found in the bronchi and spreads early to the mediastinal lymph nodes. It is very much related to smoking and will typically be preceded by progressive metaplasia caused by the constant irritation followed by constant repair, leading eventually to carcinogenic changes. It may be further categorised as keratinising or nonkeratinising.

ADENOCARCINOMA

Adenocarcinoma arises from the mucus-secreting glands of the lungs and is more often found in the peripheral parts of the lungs. It is the most common type of lung cancer, which again is related to tobacco smoking and early to metastasise.

LARGE CELL CARCINOMA

Large cell carcinoma is derived from epithelial cells but different to other categories because of their large size. It is a heterogeneous group of undifferentiated tumours and serves almost as a catch-all for anything that does not fall into other categories – a classification of exclusion.

A point of note: Lung cancer does not have to work hard to metastasise. The physiology of the lung means that malignant cells can be easily and quickly disseminated. Regardless of the type of lung cancer, many patients will present with metastases.

BOX 11.1 CLASSIFICATION OF LUNG CANCER

SMALL CELL (~18%)	NON–SMALL CELL (~80%)		
Small Cell (Oat Cell)	**Squamous Cell (~30%)**	**Adenocarcinoma (~40%)**	**Large Cell (~9%)**
• Aggressive, early metastasis • Derived from neuroendocrine cells • May secrete antidiuretic hormone, adrenocorticotrophic hormone	• Associated with smoking • Keratinising vs nonkeratinising	• Mucus-secreting glands	• Category of exclusion

Biomarkers

Various genetic aberrations can be detected in lung cancer, some of which may aid a more targeted treatment approach. Small cell lung cancers tend to be associated with inactivation of two key tumour suppressor genes, *TP53* and *RB*, leading to a failure to detect deoxyribonucleic acid (DNA) damage, and therefore unregulated cell cycle progression and may explain the rapid nature of this disease.

Non–small cell lung cancer, on the other hand, may be related to aberrations in cell growth and proliferation genes and proteins. Around 10% to 15% of NSCLCs with demonstrated mutations and amplifications is the epidermal growth factor receptor (EGFR) responsible for growth and proliferation signals to the cell. Also, around 20% to 30% of adenocarcinomas will have mutations in the *KRAS* protooncogene, which is often associated with more aggressive disease and a poorer prognosis. A small percentage of NSCLCs will be associated with the *EML4/ALK (echinoderm microtubule-associated protein-like 4 (EML4)/anaplastic lymphoma kinase (ALK))* fusion gene. This is a particular subset for which the targeted drug crizotinib (Xalkori) has been designed.

Clinical Features

Patients may present with a variety of symptoms that indicate local, lymphatic, or blood-borne spread. Local spread can involve adjacent lung tissue and give rise to respiratory symptoms, such as dyspnoea (shortness of breath), haemoptysis (bloodstained sputum) or infection. Invasion of adjacent organs by the tumour may occur, and pleural involvement may cause effusion. Invasion at the apex of the lung may cause pain to radiate down the arm, especially if there is involvement of the brachial nerve plexus, often referred to as Pancoast syndrome. Involvement of the recurrent laryngeal nerve may cause hoarseness. Involvement of mediastinal nodes, either directly or via lymphatic spread, may result in SVCO with associated swelling of the head and neck and engorgement of veins. SVCO is one of the few situations when emergency radiotherapy is called for. Other presenting symptoms may be the result of metastatic spread. Lung tumours tend to spread readily via the blood to brain, bone and liver. Eighty percent of small cell tumours will present with metastatic disease.

Staging

The TNM staging (see Chapter 1) for lung cancer is mainly based on the size of the tumour, with T1 indicating a tumour 3 cm or less, whilst T4 would mean a tumour larger than 7 cm is invading other prescribed structures. Careful assessment of lymphatic involvement is required, and the involvement of ipsilateral (same side) or contralateral (opposite side) nodes will impact on the N stage. Although TNM staging also applies to all lung cancers, the aggressive nature of small cell carcinoma and the fact that most patients present with occult metastases render the TNM staging for this disease largely unemployable. Generally, small cell carcinoma is categorised into limited disease (confined to the one hemithorax) and mediastinal and ipsilateral node involvement or extensive disease with distant metastases. As suggested earlier, many patients, regardless of the type, will present with stage IV disease.

Treatment

Small cell carcinoma: Chemotherapy is the cornerstone of any treatment for these patients. Combination chemotherapy, generally with platinum-based drugs, such as cisplatin, alongside, for example, etoposide, seems to give better results than single-agent treatment but is also associated with higher levels of treatment morbidity. For patients with limited disease, local radiotherapy may be used as an adjunct to the chemotherapy. Surgery is not recommended because of the high incidence of metastatic spread at the time of diagnosis.

Non–small cell lung cancer: In non–small cell lung cancer (NSCLC), results of standard treatment are poor in all but the most localised of cancers. Full assessment of the patient will determine whether surgery is an option. If the tumour is resectable, surgery would be the principal type of treatment. If surgery is not feasible, radical or palliative radiotherapy is the next option. Again, chemotherapy with platinum-based drugs in combination with other drugs may be used.

Radical surgery, lobectomy or pneumonectomy is the only real hope of cure for patients with small, localised tumours, but only about one-third of patients are eligible.

Radical radiotherapy should be considered for those patients in whom surgery is contraindicated but only if the disease is localised. It is only suitable for a few patients. Palliative radiotherapy is helpful in relieving symptoms. Small doses can substantially improve patients' quality of life.

For those patients with EGFR-positive disease, EGFR-directed therapies, such as gefitinib (Iressa) or erlotinib (Tarceva), may be used alongside chemotherapy, and, as stated earlier, patients with *EML4/ALK*-positive disease may be offered crizotinib (Xalkori).

Checkpoint inhibitor drugs, such as nivolumab (Opdivo), are now available as an alternative to traditional chemotherapy for patients with advanced metastatic lung cancer.

Prognosis

Despite treatment, the prognosis for lung cancer in general is very poor. Fig. 11.2 shows the 5-year survival and demonstrates the fact that most patients will present with late-stage disease (stage III or IV).

Detection of early-stage disease, although uncommon, will lead to better survival, with around 55% of patients alive after 5 years. The continued poor survival for lung cancer and a recognition that many patients present with late stage have led to attempts to try diagnosing lung cancer at an earlier stage via screening. Although no national screening programme for lung cancer exists, it continues to be investigated, with clinical trials indicating that high-risk patients (heavy or long-time smokers) could have cancer diagnosed early. However, questions still persist around overdiagnosis leading to overtreatment and cost.

THE PLEURA

At this point, it is worth mentioning the pleura. Although not part of the lung itself, the pleural cavity plays an important role in respiration and is host to an important form of malignant tumour. The pleural cavity consists of two layers of membrane. The parietal layer lines the inside of the ribs and the superior surface of the diaphragm and partitions the mediastinum. The visceral layer of the pleura, a separate pleural sac,

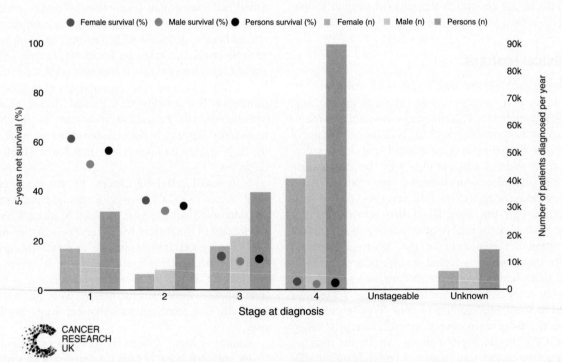

Fig. 11.2 Lung cancer 5-year survival by stage at presentation. (Source: Cancer Research UK. https://www.cancerresearchuk.org/health-professional/cancer-statistics/statistics-by-cancer-type/lung-cancer/survival#heading-Three. Accessed June 2022.)

covers the outer surface of the lung and encases each lung. The parietal and visceral layers are separated by a space containing a small amount of serous fluid that aids lubrication, thus allowing friction-free movement between the lungs and thoracic cavity on breathing.

Although the pleurae are not lung tissue, because of their close relationship, pleural and lung tumours are often grouped together. Malignant tumours of the pleura are primarily mesotheliomas. Mesothelioma is linked directly with exposure to asbestos, particularly blue asbestos; however, presentation of the disease often takes many years. At diagnosis, the tumour tends to be widespread throughout the pleural cavity. This is a direct result of transcoelomic spread throughout the serous fluid. Prognosis is difficult to determine because there is wide variation in the time before diagnosis and progression of the disease.

Localised disease is treated mainly with surgery, with extrapleural pneumonectomy offering the best chance of recurrence-free survival. Treatment for extensive disease is rarely curative, although radiotherapy can offer palliation of symptoms.

SELF-ASSESSMENT QUESTIONS

Answer true or false to the following. Answers are on page 165–166.

1 *The left lung is divided into three lobes.*

2 *SVCO is often an early sign of lung cancer.*

3 *Lung cancer is the most common form of cancer in the United Kingdom.*

4 *Smoking is implicated in all lung cancer cases.*

5 *Overexposure to passive smoke is thought to increase the risk of lung cancer in those people who do not smoke.*

6 *Adenocarcinoma of the lung often secretes antidiuretic hormone (ADH) and adrenocorticotrophic hormone (ACTH).*

7 *NSCLC refers to nonsquamous cell lung cancer.*

8 *Small cell lung cancer is often referred to as 'oat' cell.*

9 *Around 10% to 15% of NSCLC with demonstrated mutations and amplifications is the epidermal growth factor receptor (EGFR).*

10 *Small cell carcinoma of the lung is usually treated with chemotherapy.*

11 *Adenocarcinoma of the lung derives from mucus secreting glands.*

12 *A small percentage of NSCLCs will be associated with the EML4/ALK fusion gene.*

13 *The T classification for lung cancer is primarily based on the size of the tumour.*

14 *T1 N0 M0 would be interpreted as a late-stage lung tumour.*

15 *Most patients will present with late-stage disease.*

16 *Herceptin is often given to those with EGFR+ve disease.*

17 *Platinum-based drugs, such as cisplatin, alongside other chemotherapy, are a common treatment for lung cancer.*

18 *Checkpoint inhibitor drugs, such as nivolumab (Opdivo), are now available as an alternative to traditional chemotherapy for patients with advanced metastatic lung cancer.*

19 *Mesothelioma often spreads transcoelomically through the pleural cavity.*

20 *Smoking causes mesothelioma.*

Skin Cancer

Chapter Outline

Objectives

By the end of this chapter, the reader should be able to:

- Describe the anatomy of the skin, with reference to the layers of the epidermis and the types of cells found in those layers.
- Outline the risk factors for skin cancer with particular reference to the role of UV radiation.
- Compare and contrast basal cell carcinoma (BCC), squamous cell carcinoma (SCC) and melanoma.
- Outline the principles of staging for melanoma and relate this to the available treatment options.
- Explain the role of BRAF inhibitors in the treatment of melanoma.

The skin is the largest and most accessible organ of the body. Together with its accessory organs – hair, nails, sweat glands and sebaceous glands and the associated blood vessels, nerves and lymphatic vessels – it is referred to as the integumentary system. The accessory organs allow the skin to carry out its functions of protecting underlying tissue, regulating temperature by excreting perspiration, preventing excessive loss of inorganic and organic materials, receiving stimuli from the environment and synthesising vitamin D.

The skin is continuous with the mucosa of the digestive, respiratory, urinary and reproductive systems at their external openings and also with the mucosa around the eye. On average, an adult has a skin surface of around 19,000 cm^2 with a thickness varying between 0.5 and 3 mm. The skin is thinner on the dorsal (back) surfaces than on the ventral (front) surfaces. The skin consists of two main parts: the epidermis and the dermis (Fig. 12.1).

The epidermis is nonvascular (contains no blood or lymphatic vessels) and consists of four or five layers of stratified epithelium (Box 12.1). Cells

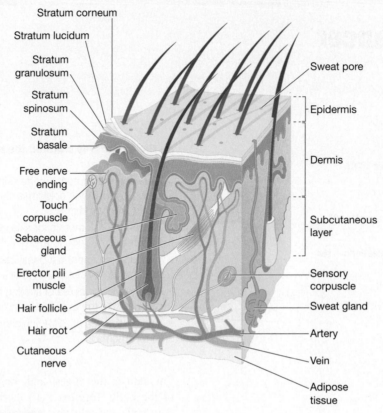

Fig. 12.1 The structure of the skin.

BOX 12.1 LAYERS OF THE EPIDERMIS

- *Stratum corneum*: 20–30 layers of flattened cells containing keratin; cells have no nuclei. This layer is continuously shed and replaced from the underlying layers. It forms a barrier to light, heat, water, chemicals and bacteria.
- *Stratum lucidum*: three to five rows of closely packed, clear, flat cells with traces of flattened nuclei; more pronounced in thicker areas of the skin, such as the palms of the hands and soles of the feet; this layer is absent in hairy skin.
- *Stratum granulosum*: three to five layers of flattening cells in which keratin is formed. Nuclear degeneration seen in this layer denotes dying cells; the keratinised cells release lipids that repel water.
- *Stratum spinosum* (prickle cell layer): 8–10 rows of polygonal cells. Melanin is taken in from the nearby melanocytes.
- *Stratum germinativum* (basal cell layer): the deepest layer; a single layer of columnar epithelium attached to a basement membrane; capable of continuous cell division and containing melanocytes.

formed from the continuous cell division of the basal layer of the epidermis gradually become more rounded and then flattened and keratinised (deposition of an insoluble protein called keratin) as they mature and rise to the surface layer. The time from cell production in the basal layer to the loss or shedding at the surface is normally 4 weeks, although in abnormal conditions such as psoriasis this can decrease to 7 to 10 days.

The dermis has two main regions: papillary and reticular. The papillary region comprises the upper 20% of the dermis and has finger-like projections called dermal papillae. It attaches the dermis to the epidermis and contains the capillaries carrying nutrients to the epidermis. Also within this layer are the sensory nerve endings for touch, pain and temperature (see Fig. 12.1). The reticular region contains denser, irregular connective tissue and contains the sebaceous and sweat glands, fat and hair follicles. The dermis, or dermal layer, provides the elasticity of the skin.

Under the dermis is a subcutaneous layer of adipose (fatty) tissue, the amount of which varies from person to person.

Melanocytes are found in the basal layer of cells and produce melanin. Skin colour is determined by the amount of the pigment melanin which infuses into the epidermal cells. Everyone has the same number of melanocytes, but differing amounts of pigment produce a range of skin colours throughout the world. Freckles are caused by patches of melanocytes; albinism is the result of having no pigment; and vitiligo is an autoimmune condition in which there is a loss of melanocytes, causing white patches. In white skin, melanin is distributed in the basal, spinosum and granulosum layers; in darker skin, it is present in all layers. When exposed to ultraviolet radiation such as that from the sun, the amount and darkness of the pigment increase, producing tanning, which gives further protection against radiation. Blood vessels in the dermis also account for some colouration, such as blushing. Carotene present in the corneum and fatty areas of the dermis along with melanin gives yellow colouring to the skin.

Oncology

Skin cancer is the most common of all malignancies worldwide but causes the fewest deaths. Incidence varies worldwide and is directly proportional to the intensity of sunlight, explaining why it is more common in Australia and South Africa than in Europe and North America. Mainly a disease of older age, skin cancer is rare under the age of 40. Malignant melanoma is more common in younger age groups than basal cell carcinoma (BCC) and squamous cell carcinoma (SCC). Overall, there is a slight male preponderance.

RISK FACTORS

The main risk factor associated with skin cancer is exposure to damaging ultraviolet (UV) radiation found in sunlight. A high percentage of skin cancers arise on exposed parts of the body, more on outdoor workers than indoor workers. People with fair skin are more prone to skin cancer because of the lack of the protective pigment melanin. Skin cancer is rare in darker-skinned populations, and when it does occur, there is an equal incidence on exposed and unexposed parts

of the body. Use of sunbeds, particularly by young people, will increase the risk of skin cancer. In countries like the UK, it is illegal for those under 18 to use sunbeds (unless for some medical reason). Other causative factors include occupational carcinogens, x-rays, immune suppression, chronic ulcers and scar tissue. Genetic factors have also been linked to skin cancer: for example, Gorlin syndrome, an autosomal dominant condition which leads to multiple BCCs, and xeroderma pigmentosum, a rare autosomal recessive disorder that predisposes the individual to SCC.

Types of Skin Cancer

The main skin cancer histologies to be considered are:
- BCC
- SCC
- melanoma.

BASAL CELL CARCINOMA AND SQUAMOUS CELL CARCINOMA

Basal Cell Carcinoma

BCC, the most common of the skin malignancies, is also referred to as a *rodent ulcer*. Histologically, there is no evidence of maturation of the cells in the epidermis from the basal layer. The cells appear uniform with darkly stained nuclei and contain little cytoplasm. Their appearance can be nodular, pigmented, sclerosing, infiltrating or ulcerative. Typically, BCC appears as a firm, pink papule with distinct raised edges and a slight depression or ulcerative centre. They normally present as a noninflammatory, painless 'spot' that becomes irritated and bleeds when scratched. BCCs are typically reported as a 'spot which does not heal'. Patients with a history of BCC should regularly check exposed skin, as multiple tumours are quite common. If left untreated, BCCs can invade locally, causing large areas of ulceration (hence the term rodent); they may destroy superficial cartilage and bone, such as that around the nose and ears, but deep invasion is uncommon, as is metastatic spread, unless they break through the basement membrane below the basal layer.

Squamous Cell Carcinoma

SCCs are less common than BCCs, even though they are associated with the same aetiolgical factors.

Histologically, they typically appear as keratinising squamous lesions in which the squamous cells penetrate the basement membrane below the basal layer and form clusters of cells in the subepithelial layer. Invasion through the basement membrane into the subepithelial layer increases the likelihood of local lymph node metastases, unlike BCCs, which tend not to penetrate this membrane. They typically appear as a crusted, scaly ulcer or an exophytic-type nodule that can be clinically difficult to distinguish from a BCC. Lesions arising at the mucocutaneous junctions tend to be more aggressive, as do those that appear in sites where the skin has been irradiated.

Staging. The TNM staging for BCC and SCC is different from that for melanoma. Essentially, it outlines the size of the tumour, with those less than or equal to 2 cm classified as stage I. Larger tumours with maybe invasion deeper beyond the subcutaneous fat would depict a later stage. Regional lymph nodes would be dictated by the location of the skin lesion.

Treatment. Lesions should be diagnosed histologically before treatment is given. This includes a biopsy that may also be the only treatment for small lesions. There are various treatments available for BCCs and SCCs, including electrocautery, cryosurgery, topical chemotherapy, excisional surgery and external beam radiotherapy. The choice of treatment depends on the site of the tumour, the cosmetic result of treatment, the availability of equipment and patient preference. All are highly effective, with around a 90% cure rate. Radiotherapy is especially useful around the eye and nose, which are difficult surgical sites, for lesions such as those on the temple and forehead, where there is less skin for surgical repair, and for large tumours that would require reconstructive surgery.

MELANOMA

Melanoma results from a malignant transformation of the melanocytes in the skin and is the deadliest form of skin cancer. It can often arise from a dysplastic nevus (changing mole) or a cluster of melanocytes, some of which can be present at birth, or may appear because of sun exposure later in life. Melanoma cancer was relatively rare in the UK prior to the 1970s, but rates have steadily increased with the advent of affordable holiday travel. Incidence varies worldwide, with Australia having an incidence much greater than that of the UK. Melanoma can affect all age groups and is directly related to levels of UV exposure, by sunlight and/or sunbeds. It is slightly more common in males, but in the 15- to 50-year-old age group it tends to be more common in women. Most melanomas will occur on exposed skin, so in women most will occur on the legs, whereas for men it occurs more frequently on the chest and back. Risk factors associated with melanoma relate to the amount, or rather the lack, of melanin; therefore, there is a higher risk for those with fair hair and freckled skin. Other risk factors include a history of severe sunburn, many moles, dysplastic nevi and a family history not connected with sun exposure. Most organs of the body have been found at post-mortem to be capable of harbouring primary melanotic foci – for example, the larynx, oesophagus and bronchi. All contain clusters of melanocytes, but why the malignant change occurs is not known.

Health education around the dangers of prolonged sun exposure has led to increased knowledge around melanoma and the increased use of UV protection.

Pathology

Melanoma will initially grow radially along the basal layer of the epidermis and if detected at this stage, before the possibility of blood vessel involvement, and then treatment is very successful. As the melanoma progresses, it will begin to invade vertically either upwards into the top layers of the epidermis or downwards into the upper part of the dermis (papillary dermis). Once this happens, the possibility of blood vessel involvement increases and so do the chances of metastatic disease. The depth of invasion is an important staging characteristic and will influence treatment options available. Melanoma is divided into cellular subtypes, each with their own characteristics, as described in Table 12.1. They include superficial spreading, nodular, lentigo maligna, acral lentiginous (palmar/plantar and subungual) and miscellaneous other cell types.

Many melanomas (around 50%) will demonstrate mutations within the BRAF [Rapidly Accelerated

TABLE 12.1	Histology of Melanoma and Characteristics		
Histology (Frequency)	**Characteristics**	**Growth Pattern**	**Body Area**
Superficial spreading (70%)	Often arise from a pigmented dysplastic nevus.	Spreads across epidermal layers before vertically.	May be found on any body surface, especially the head, neck and trunk of males and the lower extremities of females.
Nodular (10%–15%)	Symmetrical and uniform; dark brown or black (may be amelanotic).	Rapid vertical growth phase.	Common on all body surfaces, especially the trunk of males.
Lentigo maligna (10%–15%)	May have areas of hypopigmentation and often are quite large.	Linear spread as well as vertical.	Found on sun-exposed areas (e.g. hand, neck).
Acral lentiginous (5%)	Equal frequency among Black and White populations.	Extremely aggressive, with rapid progression from the radial to vertical growth phase.	Occur on the palms, soles and subungual areas (under a nail).
Other sites	Eyes, mucosa, gastrointestinal tract and genitourinary tract		

Fibrosarcoma (RAF), a family of 3 protein kinases, ARAF, BRAF & CRAF that influence cell progression and proliferation] signalling protein, which is part of the Ras, Raf, Mek, Erk signalling pathway (see Chapter 1). Such mutations render the signalling pathway permanently on, thus encouraging continued proliferation and growth of these malignant cells. Targeted therapies against the BRAF protein, such as vemurafenib (Zelboraf) and dabrafenib (Tafinilar), might be used for patients with disease which has spread. However, resistance to these drugs might ensue, usually because the cancer cell will use ARAF or CRAF signalling proteins to convey the growth signal or the MEK signalling protein may also become mutated. In such cases MEK inhibitor drugs like trametinib (Mekinist) may also be used.

Staging

Melanoma is primarily staged using the TNM system and relates to the vertical thickness of the melanoma, usually ascertained by excisional biopsy. The extent of local and distant spread is closely related to the prognosis; therefore, it is important that the stage of the disease be carefully evaluated before treatment is discussed.

The T classification is often a 'pathological' stage (p), with 1 mm or less depicting a pT1 and a lesion with thickness greater than 4 mm depicting a pT4. If there is no ulceration of the lesion, this is annotated with 'a', whilst with ulceration will be annotated with 'b'. For example, a melanoma which is 2 mm thick with ulceration would be pT2b.

The number of lymph nodes in the N staging is now used rather than the size of the nodes involved and will be dictated by the site of the primary tumour. Sentinel node biopsies may be used to help determine the possible sites for lymphatic spread. Lymph node involvement may be classed as micrometastases if it is clinically undetectable or macrometastases if it is clinically detectable.

The M staging has been subdivided to include the anatomic site of the metastases and the level of serum lactate dehydrogenase (LDH). Any M category will therefore be annotated with (0) if LDH is not elevated or (1) if LDH is elevated.

Diagnosis and Treatment

Surgery is the treatment of choice for malignant melanoma, followed by chemotherapy with or without targeted therapy. For early-stage melanoma, excisional biopsy with wide margins is usually the only required treatment with regular follow-up. For melanoma for which there is evidence of

metastases, chemotherapy in the form of dacarbazine might be offered. More likely, BRAF and
MEK inhibitor drugs (see above) will be used. The
use of checkpoint inhibitor drugs like nivolumab
(Opdivo) and ipilimumab (Yervoy) may be seen as an
alternative.

Prognosis

Prognosis is closely linked to the stage of the tumour
at presentation, and it is a case of early diagnosis saves
lives. Patients with early-stage lesions have a 5-year
survival rate of around 95%, dropping to 50% if the
lesion is over 4 mm in thickness.

SELF-ASSESSMENT QUESTIONS

Answer true or false to the following. Answers are on page 165–166.

1 *Hairy skin has the same number of epidermal layers as nonhairy skin.*

2 *The number of melanocytes gives skin its colour.*

3 *The skin comprises of a superficial dermis and deeper epidermis.*

4 *UV exposure is the most important risk factor for skin cancer.*

5 *Tumours arising at the junction of the skin and mucosa tend to be more aggressive.*

6 *A rodent ulcer is another name for a squamous cell carcinoma.*

7 *Basal cell carcinomas (BCCs) normally present as a noninflammatory 'spot that does not heal'.*

8 *Multiple BCCs are uncommon.*

9 *BCCs do not commonly metastasise.*

10 *Squamous cell carcinomas (SCCs) are less common than BCCs.*

11 *SCCs do not penetrate the basement membrane.*

12 *All melanomas are malignant.*

13 *Malignant melanomas are more common nearer the equator.*

14 *Malignant melanomas affect younger age groups than other skin cancers.*

15 *Fair-haired people are at less risk of developing malignant melanoma.*

16 *Mutated BRAF is often associated with melanoma.*

17 *The thickness of a malignant melanoma is related to the prognosis.*

18 *Surgery is the treatment of choice for malignant melanoma.*

19 *Patients with early-stage melanoma have an excellent prognosis.*

20 *Malignant melanomas spread via the lymphatics.*

ANSWERS TO SELF-ASSESSMENT QUESTIONS

Chapter 1

1. F	2. F	3. F	4. F	5. T
6. F	7. F	8. T	9. F	10. T
11. T	12. F	13. F	14. T	15. F
16. F	17. T	18. T	19. T	20. F

Chapter 2

1. F	2. F	3. T	4. T	5. T
6. F	7. F	8. T	9. T	10. T
11. F	12. F	13. T	14. F	15. F
16. T	17. T	18. F	19. T	20. F

Chapter 3

1. T	2. F	3. T	4. F	5. T
6. F	7. T	8. F	9. T	10. T
11. T	12. T	13. F	14. T	15. T
16. F	17. F	18. T	19. F	20. T

Chapter 4

1. T	2. F	3. T	4. F	5. F
6. F	7. T	8. T	9. T	10. T
11. F	12. T	13. T	14. T	15. F
16. F	17. T	18. T	19. T	20. T

Chapter 5

1. F	2. T	3. T	4. F	5. F
6. T	7. T	8. F	9. T	10. F
11. T	12. F	13. F	14. T	15. T
16. T	17. F	18. T	19. F	20. T

Chapter 6

1. F	2. T	3. F	4. T	5. T
6. F	7. T	8. T	9. F	10. T
11. T	12. F	13. T	14. T	15. F
16. T	17. T	18. F	19. T	20. F

Chapter 7

1. T	2. F	3. T	4. T	5. T
6. T	7. F	8. T	9. F	10. T
11. F	12. T	13. F	14. T	15. F
16. T	17. F	18. T	19. T	20. T

Chapter 8

1. T	2. F	3. T	4. T	5. T
6. T	7. F	8. T	9. T	10. T
11. F	12. T	13. F	14. T	15. F
16. F	17. F	18. T	19. F	20. T

Chapter 9

1. F	2. T	3. T	4. T	5. F
6. T	7. T	8. T	9. T	10. T
11. F	12. T	13. T	14. F	15. T
16. T	17. T	18. F	19. F	20. F

Chapter 11

1. F	2. F	3. F	4. F	5. T
6. F	7. F	8. T	9. T	10. T
11. T	12. T	13. T	14. F	15. T
16. F	17. T	18. T	19. T	20. F

Chapter 10

1. F	2. T	3. T	4. F	5. T
6. F	7. F	8. F	9. T	10. F
11. F	12. F	13. T	14. T	15. F
16. F	17. T	18. F	19. F	20. F

Chapter 12

1. F	2. F	3. F	4. T	5. T
6. F	7. T	8. F	9. T	10. T
11. F	12. T	13. T	14. T	15. F
16. T	17. T	18. T	19. T	20. T

Index

Note: Page numbers followed by '*f*' indicate figures and '*t*' indicate tables.